S.O.S!

Success Over Stress
For the Modern Day (Anti-Aging) Mom in Motion
Plus The Motivating Makeover Manual

Tips, Tricks, and Techniques to Manage Stress &
Augment Your Natural Beauty

By: Philippe SHOCK Matthews
Former Beauty Editor for Upscale Magazine

Foreword By: Joey Mills
(Author: New Classic Beauty)

Featuring exclusive interviews with former Essence Magazine Editor, Susan L. Taylor, Public Relations Maven, Terrie Williams, Ann Bennett Nesby, Bertice Berry, Makeup Artist, Byron Barnes, Ce Ce Peniston, Cherrelle, Cindy Herron of En Vogue, Cree Summer, Dawnn Lewis, Makeup Artist for Prince, Deborah Lake, Dr. Cheryl Burgess of Black Opal, Iman Abdulmajid, Makeup Artist, Joey Mills, Karyn White, Karyn Parsons, Lisa Fischer, Lisa Canning, Mavis Staples, Patrice Rushen, Rolonda Watts, Makeup Artist, Sam Fine, Tina Lifford, Makeup Artist Troy Jensen, Superstar, Gladys Knight, Sex Therapists, Dr. Gwendolyn Goldsby Grant, En Vogue, Yolanda Adams, and many more!

Other Books by
Philippe SHOCK Matthews:

The Shock Wealth System:
Developing the Mindset to Be Rich Before Becoming Rich

The Shock Philosophy:
A Mindset for Massive Manifestation

Shock Theology:
The Dark Side of New Thought Metaphysics & Religious Science

How to Make Millions When Thousands Have Been Laid Off:
Featuring Stedman Graham

My Four Fathers:
Personal Virtual Interviews with the Worlds Greatest Motivators Who Inspired A Fatherless Son! Featuring: Zig Ziglar | Les Brown | Brian Tracy | Dr. Denis Waitley

DEDICATION

This work is dedicated to the memory of my mother and the support and strength of my dear sister. All that I am, I owe to the both of you.

FOREWORD

One of the most critical and beneficial rituals a woman can do for her inner beauty upon awakening in the morning (before she hits the floor running) is to try to use the first moments to focus on just being quiet-through meditation, reflection, or some gentle yoga and stretching movements. This period is probably the only time during the day when uninterrupted calm is possible before one's daily obligations, work and time constraints must be faced. In the work-a-day environment there is rarely any time to focus on calm. These days each free moment has to be utilized for several things at once, doing things one at a time is a trend of the past.

In each morning there has to be ten minutes set aside to pull herself together physically and psychologically. When she feels pulled together inwardly, it's time to pamper the outer beauty too. What she is trying to do is build more presence through the confidence gained from self awareness and improved beauty due to not only the actual color imparted but the increase in self confidence that comes with improved appearance as well.

After her toilette, an efficient makeup system should be devised to fit into her tight schedule before leaving for work- a total color makeup should take less than ten minutes to apply. Makeup is an integral accessory which can heighten one's essential outer beauty and can make one feel and look more confident and natural.

Away from home to a simple makeup system is preferred, ideally with easily portable cosmetics. My own makeup system, the Joey Mills System, is based on this same concept, so that a "quick fix" touchup is possible when needed. Women need makeup designed to be put on quickly and easily portable so that whenever they find an extra ten minutes they have what they need to take advantage of it. Sometimes these precious "spare" moments freshening up in places like the office, riding in a taxi or in the restroom of a chic new club also allow time to be "quiet" again to recharge the psyche and body and shed some stress.

In today's hectic and competitive environment, feeling and looking one's best is so very important to health and success too, that the use and application of makeup, handled properly, can sometimes positively change one's outlook.

Joey Mills
(Author: New Classic Beauty)

TABLE OF CONTENTS

INTRODUCTION

She's a housewife, a working mother, an account executive, a self-employed business owner, she's you...a working woman who defies age and gravity! A woman searching for an internal beauty system and stress-free lifestyle that can handle the new workloads put on today's modern woman.

With your hectic schedule, you have to search for cosmetics and skin care products that will not only enhance your self-image but add to the efficiency of your morning schedule.

You will learn how to meditate and relax with Former Essence Magazine Editor Susan L. Taylor; how to control your thoughts with Essence Magazine Columnist, Dr. Gwendolyn Goldsby Grant; how to empower your time with Public Relations Pundit, Terrie M. Williams; and learn the powerful difference between meditation and prayer and how can use affirmations to begin and end your day.

The cosmetics industry boasts over 500 companies with an excess of 20,000 products in the marketplace! Skin care products are projected to increase about five percent per year, while lipstick, blush, eyeshadow and other items that color the face is projected to increase at ten percent per year; that's a lot of products for today's working woman to choose from.

Minimal makeup is a must these days. Speed not greed is the new makeup motto. And so if you are like many of the women who fit the above profile, you apply your makeup every morning on the run. While eating a bagel, while in the ladies lounge, on the bus, plane or train or in your car between go lights. Dabbing lipstick here, and sweeping eyeshadow there; these are the places where you make the effort to project a positive self-image. But don't you find it difficult and stressful trying to make it through the montage of products, applications and techniques that are essential for projecting a positive self-image?

Well that is why this book is dedicated to empowering your self-image and giving you effective methods of applying your cosmetics and skin care in the morning to accommodate your active lifestyle. These days most cosmetics are generally problem-free, there are strict controls on ingredients, labeling and safety tests. And provided they are applied correctly, makeup can have a dramatic effect on the way you look and feel about yourself, improving your overall self-identity.

You'll enjoy chapters that will address the importance of deflecting stress and preparing your mind for the day ahead. I think this is the most important component to any woman's day. Throughout my years of makeup artistry, interviewing image-conscious entertainers, and being an internet empowerment trainer, I've come to realize that women needed to not only know how to apply their makeup, but they also need to know the proper attitude in which to apply it.

Meditation, visualization and affirmation are three mental ingredients you'll be introduced to first. When blended together, these principles will ensure peace of mind, calmness and sound self-esteem in the midst of all your daily duties.

I really hope you enjoy the plethora of information of I have included in the chapters dedicated to eliminating stress and preparing your mind for the day's activities. I know that it is hard for every woman to go about tasks and still manage to think about themselves. However, I also believe that having "me-time" is essential in making your day a whole lot better. And these chapters on stress management and daily preparations will serve as your guide to make your life free from stress.

Whether you're a working mother or a stay at home mom, you need to know the techniques to reduce stress. A life lived that is filled with stress is not a good thing, and this book is here to teach you how to banish this from your life.

One of the best tips highlighted for women is the power of meditation. Taking time out just to breathe and relax helps alleviate all your tensions. Through the art of meditation, you'll find that all your worries vanished from existence and feel like a really heavy load has been lifted off of you.

Given that it's been practised for thousands of years, it's no wonder why it is still an effective form of relaxation and stress reduction. By simply clearing your mind of everything that's been bothering you, you can enhance both your physical and mental well-being. Now, isn't that what you want?

In this book, you will find tips you need on meditation which includes advice on creating a meditative atmosphere. Another interesting activity related to relaxation is yoga, and this book features tips on yoga breathing.

A chapter focusing solely on visualization is also provided. Visualization is a very powerful tool and when used in conjunction with meditation can produce really great results. Visualization is basically picturing what you want to get in your mind. You can visualize your ideal holiday: on a quiet island, lying on a hammock and reading a good book with the sound of waves lapping on the shore and the sun smiling happily on you.

This same visualization can be done with your entire work day. Rather than think about what a stressful day will be right ahead of you, fill your mind with positive thoughts and these will make your day a whole lot better. And the chapter dedicated solely to visualization will help you do exactly that.

In that chapter, you will learn how to visualize an inner sanctuary. This will be your "safe haven" or your "happy place" if you will. This is where you can escape to when you feel the pressures of the day mounting on you. It is a temporary relief so that you don't go mad about deadlines and such. Rather than react, retract. Go into a place where you feel safe and you'll totally feel a whole lot better afterwards. And most importantly, ready to move on to the next challenge.

Having written about creating an inner sanctuary where you can run off to when things go bad, I also provide a chapter on affirmations. Everyone needs positive encouragement to know that they have done the right thing. They need affirmations from the people they love and trust to get on with the day. However, there are also affirmations of the personal kind.

Yes, I believe every woman should make it a habit to affirm themselves positively each and every day. Simply telling yourself to "love yourself more every waking moment" does a lot for your spirit. It's self-empowerment that will help drive your self-esteem way high.

Ladies, having a high self-esteem isn't bad at all. Every woman needs to be confident of who she is – in and out. She needs to be happy about herself no matter her body size, no matter how much she weighs. It's important for women to feel that and you can achieve this with the internal dialogue you make with yourself.

It's these internal conversations that you make that will bring out only the best in you. And when you have created some really good affirmations for yourself, it will show on the outside. People will notice a different level of aura to you. Positive internal reinforcements just makes you bloom.

Of course, the chapter on affirmations will teach you everything you need to know about how you can encourage yourself through thought and inner conversations. It teaches you how to write your own affirmations as a technique to improve self-confidence. After all, having a positive self-image will boost your confidence levels and will help you succeed in whatever challenges you have to face during the day.

This book is designed to help with stress relief for mothers, be they a single mother or an entrepreneurial mother.

Of course, once you have pulled yourself together on a mental level, it's now time to paint the exterior canvas of your being. Yes, this means it's time to think about your outer appearance. I know that it's hard for women to find a look that works each and every day, but there are simple tips and tricks that make it a whole lot easier to paint that blank canvas.

I have provided chapters on how to do makeup properly. I believe that you shouldn't do too much to your face. There is elegance in simplicity and it will show. For example, you don't need to pair a really catchy shade of lipstick with an equally attention-grabbing eye shadow. Balance is a key in executing the perfect makeup, and I have put together lots of information on helping you achieve a really balanced look. It's filled with a whole lot of tips, including foundation, concealer, powder, eyeliner and more to have a really harmonious look.

There's a chapter on the basics of developing good skin care habits, where you'll hear what actress Karyn Parsons and singer Karyn White have to say about the simplicities of their skin care routine. You'll discover what products I highly recommend for quick, yet efficient skin cleansing, toning and moisturizing products on the market. And you'll find out what the most important ingredient in maintaining a healthy, radiant glow to your skin is.

It is also important to note that you have to recognize your uniqueness to be able to appreciate your beauty. As what I've said in The Shock Wealth System book, *"YOU ARE UNIQUE AND UNREPEATABLE: Accept the fact that you are unique and different. If you've ever been labeled odd, crazy or eccentric, realize that you are a genius. Public relations pundit Terrie Williams said, If you're feeling a little bit weird, or out of place, not to worry. It means you are destined for great things! No amount of not fitting in will stand in the way of your path to success if you don't let it."*

Throughout the book, you'll be introduced to Special Quick Tips such as the effects of Aromatherapy and music to support your morning meditation process. Timeless and ageless beauties such as Cindy Herron of En Vogue, Ce Ce Peniston, Rolonda Watts, Cherrelle, and public relations diva Terrie Williams will share with you their quick tip beauty secrets for stress-free mind, body and spirit. Susan L. Taylor of will even share her morning meditation ritual and supermodel/actress Iman will teach women of color the importance of matching foundation and choosing a good face powder.

Celebrity Makeup Artist's such as Joey Mills, Byron Barnes, Sam Fine and Deborah Lake will lend a few of their tricks of the trade and image enhancement advice to fortify your image regime. Plus you'll find over 30 Quick Tips to speed you through your meditation, skincare and makeup process and be introduced to my Quick Pix of cosmetics companies and products that I recommend for the woman in motion.

Of course, starting your day right isn't the only thing that matters. How you end your day is also a big thing. It's important to start your day on a good note and end it on an even better one. And yes, capping off your day with bright cheer does have a lot to do with being able to relax.

And I have a section dedicated to how you can relax after a day at work or however you spent an entire day. I share relaxation activities that you can do in order to make the end a stressful day and make it a whole lot better. No matter the troubles of the day, it's best to leave them where they belong: in the past. The end of the day is time for you to regroup, recharge and prepare for a new challenge that lies ahead.

This book will teach you how to reduce stress and feel fabulous with the right relaxation, skin care and makeup techniques. I hope you do enjoy the journey.

Enjoy!

PART 1

IN THE MORNING: MEDITATION TO GET YOU GOING

Quiet Time: Feeling The Calm Before The Storm

You awake abruptly to the buzzing, ringing, annoying sound of your alarm clock. Your heart races as you realize the house isn't burning down, but you have to get up-another work day. You gather your thoughts and realize you have a high pressured day awaiting you, so you begin anticipating all of the things that could go wrong for the day, because most of the same things happened yesterday. As your mind continues this forecast of failure, you begin getting agitated and angry because you now have to get up and partake once again in this madness called your job! You put one foot on the floor, then the other. You scratch your head, and other accouterments, smack your mouth and release a smidgen of morning breath that unwillingly greets your nose.

Does this sound familiar to you? If so, it's far time that you make a commitment to change your attitude about how you begin your day. Why? Because it's vital for you to realize the importance of quiet time, and feeling the calm before the storm. Unfortunately, most women begin their day jumping out of bed, into the shower, wolfing down a bagel, running hither and dither, and never giving themselves a chance to harness a harmony that could rule the entire pace of their day. If you're like most working women, this need to slow down and catch your breath is all too real but seemingly impossible.

A Woman And Her Stress

"I will not stand for mediocrity under no circumstances! I would never compromise on that."

- Terrie Williams

New York-based, Public Relations Diva Terrie Williams, and Author of "The Personal Touch", is known in her industry as the Princess of PR, she is one such woman who fits all counts of the aforementioned.

Terrie heads The Terrie Williams Agency, a million dollar plus conglomerate made up of journalists, marketing, media relations and publicity specialists, all skilled at publicizing such clients as Anita Baker, Sally Jessy Raphael, Jackie Joyner-Kersey, Hammer, Eddie Murphy, the late Johnnie Cockeran and Janet Jackson.

Terrie knows stress all too well as her days multiply into a frenetic lifestyle that has driven her to be the best in her field. She drives her company to be the very best in the industry by not giving in to her personal pet peeve -- mediocrity. She's so adamant about being the best, she once told me in an interview:

I will not stand for mediocrity under no circumstances! I would never compromise on that. I have very, very high standards. I'm very demanding of Terrie, and anybody that's on my team. I think you have to go through life giving a hundred percent, and to say that you're serious about something, I expect you to be above average, to stand out, to have integrity, and to care about the people around you that you work with and the world at large.

Terrie begins her day with a morning walk around New York's Jacqueline Kennedy Onassis reservoir in Central Park to mentally prepare herself for the day that awaits. Once she gets to the office at seven or eight o'clock, she spends an hour of her morning devoted to what she refers to as "skim reading," where she reads an average of six newspapers a day with the aid of one of her junior assistants. *"We read several newspapers a day here at the agency," Terrie says. "Because it's imperative. You've gotta' know who's doing what with whom. What's in there about your clients and how it may impact on them or what kinds of issues you might need to respond to for the day."*

Terrie is most determined about staying on top of her information driven industry. She protects her morning mind-meld with vigilance, allowing nothing to interrupt her regimen. *"I don't like to do anything before I read my newspapers,"* she admits. *"People know that's my quiet time, because once the phone starts ringing, and I start answering, and dealing with inquiries, I get too easily distracted."* In fact, Terrie is so devoted to her reading ritual, during her book signing tour, she described having gotten to bed at 1:30 in the morning the night her book was launched in New York with a 6:30 a.m. flight to Chicago the next day. She says, *"I was really, really tired, but I had to read the newspapers on my way to the airport!"*

But her devotion doesn't stop there; on Sunday's Terrie says, *"I go to my out of town newsstand and get the LA Times, and the Washington Post, then I go through another fifty sections of newspapers. It's important to be well informed, if you're going to be exceptional at what you do."* Terrie believes that above average behavior is the only key to unlocking a successful business, something that she makes sure her team knows all too well. "I expect those things from anybody that is on my team, and if you don't strive for those things, then I respect the fact that you should go work somewhere else, but not here!"

Harsh as this may sound, for many women running their own businesses, or who are in top level management, or even running their own household, the Terrie Williams discipline happens to be a daily reality! If this is you, it is important for you to make a deliberate and determined effort in finding balance and serenity for the day that awaits you.

Don't Hesitate...Meditate

Morning meditation is fast becoming a staple in the way many women begin their diurnal duties. Eastern religions such as Hinduism, Buddhism, Taoism and Islamic Sufism have used meditation as a path to enlightenment for centuries. If you believe that your thoughts affect the things that you experience in life, then you'll understand the importance of finding quiet moments of peace and stillness before plunging into your day.

Here's one great example of how helpful meditation is excerpted from The Shock Wealth System:

[BEGIN EXCERPT]

One of Chicago's top radio talk show hosts, Ty Wansley came under the dark cloud of other people's opinions when he began feeling the daily pressures of drinking and drugs associated with the entertainment business. Ty told me: I don't drink, I don't smoke, and I don't do narcotics, and it seemed when I started in the business everybody was doing dope. If you didn't do dope, you [were] considered a square, and I didn't want to be perceived as a square, but doing dope is stupid!

Ty fought back, not relinquishing his power to someone else's negativity and a negative environment. Instead he practiced "TM" or Transcendental Meditation, taught to him by Stevie Wonder's ex-wife, Sarita Wright. She seemed so spiritual, Ty recalled. I was going through all of this turmoil about people telling me, 'You've got to do dope!' They wanted me to do all of these trappings and diversions. I sensed serenity and peacefulness with Sarita, and I was always fascinated by the concept of meditation. Since that moment in his life, Ty has been meditating twice a day ever since and it has kept him focused away from the negative words, thoughts and actions of other people's opinions of him.

[END EXCERPT]

Susan L. Taylor, is another working woman who must juggle the role of mother, wife and editor of Essence magazine, along with the celebrity that comes from promoting her books. Her day begins at 5:30 in the morning with a hot bath, laced with fragrant oils and surrounded by scented candles while listening to a meditation tape. She then affirms what she's going to accomplish for the day ahead, and after about 30 minutes of exercise and a sprightly walk, she leaps into her day of meetings, editing, and presentations. *"We have to take what I call quiet time," she says. "Press away from the world. It's not about mantras, prayers and rote incantations, it's about being still and allowing that still small voice within you express itself and to give you guidance and direction. When we do that consistently, we feel strong and when the crisis comes, it may knock us down, but it doesn't knock us out, cause we know that there's something inside of us that is stronger than any adversity outside of us."*

This still small voice that Susan speaks of has often been referred to as the voice of God or Divine Intuition. Whatever this method of relaxation presents itself, meditation is one of the most powerful means of bringing an inner peace to a restless mind plagued by the noises of the world. What all meditation has in common is that it produces a deep state of relaxation and self-assurance, which rejuvenates both mind and body. The aim of meditation is to free the mind of all disturbing thoughts and to remain in a state of restfulness while fully alert.

The Difference Between Meditation And Prayer

A key fact about meditation is that it can be adapted into any faith or religion, since there is a distinct difference between meditation and prayer as there is a distinct difference between religion and spirituality. In traditional times, prayer was viewed and taught as asking for desires and answers to a problem or crisis. Contemporary techniques of meditation teaches you just to affirm in your mind what it is you want, and behave in a manner as if your desire has already been manifested.

Susan explained that, *"Religion and spirituality are different. Religion has to do with ritual-going to the church, going to the mosque, going to the synagogue. Its genuflecting, getting down on your knees and saying prayers. Spirituality means living and breathing the truth of who you are and trying to be aware of it, that we are not just flesh, blood and bones, there is a holy spirit that resides in each one of us, and we really don't learn that in the school, or in church."*

There are a sundry of books on the subject of meditation. Although the effects of meditation is vastly different for each individual, finding your own groove is a matter of practice and individual experimentation. Author and lecturer of several books on the subject of meditation Sri Chinmoy remarked in his book entitled Meditation: Man-Perfection in God-Satisfaction, *"It is only through meditation that we can get lasting peace, divine peace. If we meditate soulfully in the morning and receive peace for only one minute, that one minute of peace will permeate our whole day. And when we have a meditation of the highest order, then we get really abiding peace, light and delight."*

Creating A Meditative Atmosphere

To create a meditative atmosphere, you want to quiet your immediate surroundings before engaging in any form of meditation. This may be difficult at first if you're a beginner, but soon it will become second nature to you. Create a meditative sanctuary first by zoning off a special room and sitting area for your journey within. Eliminate environmental distractions like the telephone, screaming children, television and radios. You may even want to go as far as putting a note on your door saying DO NOT DISTURB FOR 15 MINUTES OR ELSE! If need be, invest in earplugs if your environment is too noisy.

Meditation works best when applied early in the morning before the rest of the minds of the world become active. A keynote I'd like to add about meditation is don't get too wrapped up in trying to hear something, or making something happen. You can't work at meditation, you just open up to the idea of it and become aware of its silence. Meditation isn't done by doing anything, its done by being.

Creating a meditative atmosphere doesn't have to be limited to just sitting in a chair in a particular room either, a meditative atmosphere can be in your shower, your bath, or even in your car before pulling out of your driveway. There are several meditative exercises to choose from, once you learn the basic techniques of meditation, you will automatically find the method or methods that best suit your needs.

QUICK TIP:

To increase your relaxation and meditation, try sprinkling two unscented dry towels with one of your favorite scents or fragrance. Lavender or vanilla are great for relaxation and meditation. Put the towels in your clothes dryer for a few minutes until they heat up, then give yourself a vigorous rubdown. The hot, fragrant towels will feel absolutely sensational against your body.

Number One: Stilling The Mind

With your eyes closed, sit quietly, relaxed with your mind fixed on the moment. Become aware of your breathing. Understand, meditation is like rhythmic breathing, providing a wonderful way to flow with the calming energy within. Take two or three deep breathes to really relax your nerves and muscles. Follow your breath in and out. There should be no tension in your body, nor should there be any worries, concerns or anxieties hovering in your mind about the day that faces you. And don't "try" to breathe, just follow your breathe as it naturally flows.

Number Two: Learning To Observe

Now that your body and mind is relaxed, you will most certainly experience what's described by many burgeoning meditator's and even some seasoned as "mental chatter." Mental chatter is where your mind races a mile a minute on non-important thoughts and concerns such as:

"What am I going to do after this is over?"
"What about the rent and car note?"
"Is this meditation stuff really working?"
"Why am I not peaceful yet?"
"Where is that still small voice the author was talking about?"

When this happens, and it will, simply do nothing, just observe it and gently dismiss it. Tell your thoughts *"I'm busy right now and have no time for you."* Don't' try and fight it, because what you resist persists. Learn to observe your thoughts. Observation is basically a meditation of acceptance, letting go and dismissing intrusive thoughts to quiet your mind. Just learn to say "no" to the mental chatter, and hold your concentration as you penetrate the "mental chatter."

Number Three: Finding Your Light

The Light has been described by many as a spiritual presence or invisible life force that responds to human thought and interaction. The Chinese call this Light Chi and practices Chi Gong, or Chinese meditation. Legendary Vocalist Gladys Knight defines the Light as spiritual beauty. She says, *"Beauty to me is spiritual. God is in everything, and God is in all of us. If we have Him with us, He's going to shine."* Seeing the Light as total beauty and pervasiveness, Gladys described the Light metaphorically. *"You know those little balls that kids use to play with? There's light on the inside and it has these holes on the outside. When you turn on the light, all the little rays of light come out, that's what I see. That's what beauty is to me, it's in the flowers, it's in people, it's all around us if we know how to pull it out."*

The Light is omnipresent. It is with you always, but is only felt in the deepest and absolute stillness of your mind and heart. Its your very own, individualized inner energy that fulfills all of your desires and wishes, and abides at the very core of your being. Light is an energy force that is greater than the debts you owe, greater than the relationships that cause you turmoil, greater than the trials and tribulations that face you in your career and life. Its a force that heals and responds only to your hope or faith in its ability to transcend and enlighten the dark areas of day-to-day living.

Number Four: Using Your Light: An Exercise In Meditation

In accessing your Light, in your mind, sense a pure, bright radiating Light representing your Life Force. Imagine it first in the center of your heart, then sense it expanding to engulf your entire body until you literally feel like you're glowing from the inside out. Feel the Light going through every vein, nerve, fiber and tissue in your body. Remember, this is a healing Light and it neither hurts nor harm anything or anyone, so you should feel complete peace, serenity and safety with a slight smile of calmness on your face. ANYTHING opposite of these feelings is not the Light and should be gently, but assuredly, dismissed. Abide in your awareness of this Light for as long as you can. Five minutes a day will soon turn into fifteen, then thirty and more.

By using meditation every morning before beginning your day, you'll begin noticing incremental shifts in how you respond to your usual stresses and pressures. Meditating with your Light doesn't change everything for you necessarily, but it does change you for everything!

"Meditation tells us only one thing; God is. Meditation reveals to us only one truth; ours is the vision of God."

- Sri Chinmoy

SPECIAL QUICK TIP: Tension, Relaxation & Breath Control

Breathing is the most vital of all survival functions and necessities; you can live without water for a week, or food for over a month, but you cannot live without oxygen and breath for more than a few minutes. Learning how to deep breathe will not only soothe your nerves, but it will revitalize your complexion as well.

When your body is tense, learn to relax and breathe deeply. This is a simple statement, but not so easy to accomplish, because there are so many culprits that causes tension and stress. Dissatisfaction, worry, frustration, fear and anger; the inability to adapt to new situations and circumstances in your environment, or boredom with your job or career-any of these symptoms individually or in combination will cause undue nervousness and tension.

Why is tension such a bad thing? Well, for one when the body is tense, fatigued, toxins build up in the body. The same kind of build up that would occur if you were to ignore a stopped up kitchen pipe. Emotional tension even blocks the normal function of your diaphragm, the muscle that regulates the lungs and heart from the abdominal cavity. That knot that you may feel in your stomach when tension flares up is actually the contracting or tightening of your diaphragm. When the diaphragm tightens, it hinders normal breathing and cuts off blood circulation to your arms and legs, and the body begins to stiffen.

Breathing, or drawing in large amounts of oxygen and exhaling carbon dioxide, purifies the blood and helps burn up the toxic waste in the body. Unfortunately, when we breathe, most of us only fill our lungs to only one-eighth of their capacity. In order to relieve stress and tension, you must learn to breathe fully and deeply, producing higher flow of oxygen which burns up large quantities of waste material in your body.

Yoga breathing in particular is effective in manifesting good habits in breath control, maximizing your lung capacity. Yoga breathing will also rectify the shallow breathing causes the body to devitalize, have low energy levels, chronic fatigue and mental depression.

Below is an exercise for Deep Yoga Breathing

1) Place both of your hands on your rib cage and exhale completely.

2) Through your nose, inhale very slowly and count to 5 until your abdomen is filled with as much air as you can stand.

3) Now go beyond and continue to inhale slowly, counting another 5 seconds and expand your chest. Do this until your chest is filled with air.

4) For a count of 5, hold the air in your chest and abdomen.

5) Very slowly, exhale through your nose to a count of 10 and with your stomach, push the air out until your lungs are emptied.

With practice, Deep Yoga Breathing should take about 25 seconds to complete. Do this exercise before your meditation in the morning or before retiring for the evening. You will find yourself having more energy, less fatigue and stress.

PART 2

IN THE MORNING: VISUALIZATION TO KEEP YOU GOING

Seeing The Calm Before The Storm

Comedian Flip Wilson use to always say, "What you see is what you get!" Visualization is a form of seeing what you want to get, a form of concentrated seeing if you will. Visualization is different from daydreaming, because daydreaming is not controlled thinking, its random, and doesn't command the power of focus. Visualization is not visual either, its emotional. Visual is seeing with your eyes, whereas visualization is seeing with your mind and heart.

Visualization is easier than it may sound, since everything you do in your day, begins with a vision or thought; you have to see what it is you want to do in some way in order to carry out the order of the thought. And what you visualize creates a new sense of reality for you as well, because what you see in your mind greatly affects your moods and emotions. Remember in Quiet Time: Feeling The Calm Before The Storm, where I explained: You awake abruptly to the buzzing, ringing, annoying sound of your alarm clock. Your heart races as you realize the house isn't burning down, but you do have to get up. You gather your thoughts and realize you have a high pressured day awaiting you? All of these thoughts are literally pictures in your mind, especially as you began planning the day ahead.

Visualization Used In Tandem With Meditation

So it would be safe to say that visualization could be the most powerful form of meditation known, especially when used in tandem with your Light in meditation. It can reveal whole new realities of calming, stress-free alternatives. When melded with meditation, visualization locks in the principle of faith, developing a kind of laser beam effect within your imagination. Visualizing gives you the power to create a new future for yourself. Focus, faith and follow-through are the three keys to locking in the daily desire for harmony. Visualization creates realization, and a realization, by default creates a manifestation of the visualization.

The late Dr. Maxwell Maltz, a renown Plastic Surgeon who taught his patients to use visualization techniques before and after cosmetic surgery in his book 'Psycho- Cybernetics', spoke profoundly on the technique of visualization explaining that your *"...Brain and nervous system cannot tell the difference between a "real" experience, and one which is vividly imagined. The possibility of the goal must be seen so clear that it becomes "real" to your brain and nervous system. So real, in fact, that the same feelings are evoked as would be present if the goal were already achieved."* The stronger your vision is of conquering your daily stresses, the stronger the feelings and emotions will be in actualizing your stress-free mentality.

Another notable personality who makes use of visualization with meditation is Les Brown. Here's how he incorporates healthy living for higher production, from the book, My Four Fathers: Personal Virtual Interviews with the Worlds Greatest Motivators Who Inspired A Fatherless Son!

To reach his own higher level of self awareness, Les's daily routine is simple yet effective -- meditation about three times a day, he doesn't drink or smoke, he exercises, avoids greasy foods, drinks a lot of water, and gets massages every week. *"I love to walk," says Les. "You must be what you talk about. I make it my business to live my message. Attitude has a lot to do with the aging process. Because, I make a conscious effort to work hard to do what I do and empower other people, if they get just a small percentage of what I get, that gives me energy. I thank God for giving me the opportunity to be an active force in the lives of people -- to help them realize things about themselves that they didn't know -- the same as someone did for me."*

Releasing Preordained Stresses Of The Day

Diligently holding a vision in your mind of peace and harmony will create a fundamental foundation of faith that alleviates preordained stress. It's creating the belief or faith that whatever it is you desire, already exists within the abiding Light within you. Understanding this principle of faith helps us to understand how traditional prayer may have transcended into modern day meditation. Remember meditation is "being" and "affirming," not asking. Besides, why would you ask for something you already have anyway? Just because you are not aware of it at the moment, does not mean it hasn't existed for you all along. You must affirm peace and harmony every day in your meditations, sensing that dream is already fulfilled!

Two books I highly recommend on the subject of visualization are Creative Visualization: Use the Power of Your Imagination to Create What You Want in Your Life by Shakti Gawain and Dynamic Thought by Henry Hamblin Thomas. Says Hamblin, *"The fact that you can see with your mind's eye that which you have created by your mental processes, is proof that what you have created exists. If it did not exist, you could not see it."* Believe in the power of your Light functioning as your desires, and you will become a beacon of Light for all of your desires to manifest through! It was Ralph Waldo Emerson said it best: *"All that I have seen teaches me to trust the Creator for all I have not seen."*

Visualizing An Inner Sanctuary

A sanctuary is an inner retreat, that you build using visualization techniques to house and use your Light. Your inner sanctuary can be any shape, size or location you feel comfortable with. Be it on a mountain top overlooking the ocean, a valley, a brook, or even a lush green garden, or floating effortlessly in space.

In creating your inner sanctuary, allow your inner awareness to help you with the design of your safe-haven, just let your imagination run wild until you have created your dream escape. You can augment the reality of your sanctuary with soft music playing while in meditation, or you can simply imagine the sound of the ocean roaring gently in the background of your mind. You can also use scents and aromas to increase your state of relaxation and visualization. Lighting scented candles or incense is one option you can use to enhance your visual senses, or you can spray your favorite fragrance.

Once you created this inner sanctuary, it will become your rock, your calm in the midst of the daily storm. It is important that this sanctuary feels safe from any negative or pessimistic intrusions, so always enter your sanctuary with your Light to protect you from the negative intrusion of mental chatter and outside influences.

Visualization/Meditation Exercise

Now as in the meditation process, with your eyes closed, sit quietly, relaxed with your mind fixed on the moment. Become aware of your breathing then allow the Light to permeate and engulf your total being as before. For the sake of this exercise, let's create a garden sanctuary. Picture yourself sitting comfortably in a lavish expansion of flowers, trees, shrubs and greenland. Feel the serenity and safety of this awe inspiring vista. Notice the birds in the trees, hear them chirping in your mind. Notice the vibrant colors of the flowers and the sweet smell they relinquish in the air around you. Notice the smoothness of the grass you're sitting or lying on, and how beautifully velvet it is.

Now deeply sense the overall harmony of this vision. See the sun illuminating the garden, and feel the sun gently warming your face and body as it represents your Light. Feel a warm soothing breeze blowing over you, and smell the collective freshness that your garden sanctuary has created for you. Abide here in your garden sanctuary for about 15 to 30 minutes a day and watch the stress disappear.

PART 3

THE MOTIVATION: AFFIRMATIONS TO ENSURE YOUR MORNING ARRIVAL

Sending Your Light

Your Light is closer to you than the air you breathe, and you can apply your Light to any area of your life that does not represent harmony and peace simply by using the power of affirmation. If you know you're going to be faced with an argumentative day, create a mental shield by speaking words of self-empowerment.

An Exercise Of Affirming

Go back into your garden sanctuary, surround yourself with Light and recreate the feeling of peace and harmony. Now gently think about the problem or concern that may be facing you this day. The problem or concern could be big or small, but just think about it without getting angered or too involved. Just notice it from a safe distance outside of your garden sanctuary, clear from its negative sting. Now envision a ray of your Light descending upon the problem, and deeply feel the peace and overcoming of the problem that your Light has zapped with its laser beam.

But don't stop here. While envisioning the peace within the problem, solidify the vision by speaking the words-an affirmation. To affirm means to make firm, grounding your thoughts, desires and visions so they appear and feel more real to you. Using affirmations is like using corrector tape on a typewriter, it self-corrects a negative situation with the Light of truth and harmonizes the dysfunction of the situation. So as you visualize overcoming this problem, say to yourself:

"I affirm the dissolving of this problem (write it out if you have to), and the restoration of peace and harmony to this situation. This or something better comes to me right now, for the highest good of all concerned."

Or,

"I bless the days events that lie ahead of me for the highest good of all concerned."

Now become aware of your breathing again, and slowly open your eyes. You should feel empowered and rejuvenated. Repeat this process at least twice daily, once in the morning and once before retiring for bed, or as many times as you feel is necessary.

Whatever the situations or problems are that face you, by using this technique of sending out your Light and affirming its solution, you will greatly diminish the emotional charges and effects of the problem. Done regularly, you will literally pre-program yourself to respond to challenges and obstacles with strength and self-assurance.

More Affirmations For A Stress-free Day

"Today is my day in every way. I am empowered, I am at peace and I hold strong of my faith in my Light."

"Everyday and in every way, I am getting better and better at what I do and how I do it."

"I am free of stress, I am free of worry and anxiety. This is my day to shine and be fine."

"I release Light on every problem, on every challenge, on every concern that faces me this day. Nothing and no one can shake my faith in my Light."

"I bless it, and I don't stress it!"

Self-empowering Affirmations

To Make You Love The Way You Look

Now that you've learned how to send out your personal Light to dispel the darkness of a stressful day, I'd like to show you how to personalize your affirmations to boost your self-esteem and your self-image.

If thoughts are the seeds of personal beliefs, then affirmations must be the fertilizer that manifest those beliefs. Affirming yourself as beautiful and attractive is not locking in a narcissus self-image, not in the least bit. In fact, it should be considered quite normal. At the very least, you should expect to be beautiful, expect to be attractive, expect to look, feel and be wonderful! Why, you might ask? Because you are wonderful, so there!

Affirming yourself is doing nothing more than stating a fact that already exist. So with or without makeup, affirm to yourself you are beautiful and attractive, right now! Please make an effort to develop a no-nonsense attitude about these facts. Remember the old admonishment: If you don't stand for something, you could fall for anything!

Creating A Positive Self-image

Affirming your beauty, especially in the beginning of your day, creates powerful motivation and what I call a "Positive Self-Image" or PSI. Affirming your beauty individualizes and defines you, helping you to discover your own uniqueness and inner beauty.

Actress Cree Summer told me once that she was still discovering her own beauty. Trying not to make any alterations, and trying to see herself with my own eyes, and not through the eyes of other people. Cree believes that beauty is self- love and self-acceptance, and says that she will *"Know true beauty when I know me."* But, a lot of women I've spoken to don't feel beautiful, especially upon awakening in the morning. With sleepy-time still in their eyes, they're grumpy because they have to get up. One woman I talked to espoused, *"The wrinkles from my pillow are still firmly etched in my face in the morning!"*

Moreover, thinking positive about your day ahead will also help you get through gracefully. By putting aside negativities right when you wake up and affirming your beauty from within, you'll be able to face the day more confidently. As discussed in My Four Fathers book, *"What you do is you start getting rid of the things in your life that are bringing you down, the negative relationships, the negative inputs and you start replacing it with the positive. You take action on that. That's how you start to build. There's a story in Atlanta, the city was moving in a direction and it was towards the landfill where all the garbage was. The city fathers knew that one day that would be like the center of the city."*

Unlike bad, morning breath, which can be washed out with mouthwash, bad attitudes in the morning are not as easy to eradicate, and usually manifest themselves as negative self-talk. Did you know that 80% of our self-dialogue is negative? You literally support self-negativity whenever you look into your mirror and say, *"I'm too fat...I hate the way I look,"* or *"My skin is horrible."* These are affirmations of disempowerment, and when spoken with belief and conviction, sabotage your self-image, creating low self-esteem and self-worth. So PLEASE, do not speak negatively of yourself, or put yourself down when in conversation with someone else-not even in fun...ok? Ok!

So here's what I want you to do. While you're in front of your makeup mirror just about to apply your skin care, foundation, powder and color, use two or three self-affirming statements to yourself and watch a natural smile of assurance spread across your face. In order to look good, you must be able to feel good about yourself, and in developing a Positive Self-Image it takes only two things: Responsibility and Discipline. Responsibility to begin everyday positively affirming yourself, and the Discipline to never stop affirming yourself throughout the course of your day for the rest of your life.

Nationally acclaimed Psychotherapist Dr. Gwendolyn Goldsby Grant, and Author of The Best Kind of Loving: A Black Woman's Guide to Finding Intimacy is very well versed in positive self-affirmation and raising self-esteem. In fact, her advice column Between Us that appears monthly in the pages of Essence Magazine gives women sound advice of all ages who may have forgotten how to emotionally and verbally take better care of themselves. I remember meeting Dr. Grant at a restaurant in Chicago when she was in town facilitating one of her "For Women Only" Seminars. I specifically asked her what can women do immediately in their lives to begin empowering their overall self-image and esteem. Here's what she told me:

Start being a self-caretaker. The first thing you have to do is get into romantic encounters with yourself. Do it with imagery. Begin to look at yourself in the mirror. Strip nude. Take off all your clothes and stand in the mirror, and begin taking apart each part of your body. Start with your hair, and go all the way down.

Then you do what is called your prayer of acceptance. Every wrinkle, every fold, every inch-accept every part of yourself. You say to yourself, my eyes are beautiful, my makeup is beautiful, everything is beautiful. Start by saying loving and endearing things to yourself, 'Good morning dear, how are you?' Do that every day.

Some good advice to say the least, and not just for women, I've tried this technique on myself and believe me it works! Talking to yourself and speaking words of self-empowerment will not only make you feel like a million bucks, it can keep you looking like a million bucks too. Age is truly a number. More than that, its a state of mind, and if your mind is stayed on negative thoughts, your words and behaviors are going to reflect that throughout your self-image. So, it doesn't matter what your weight, height, or economic status is, what matters is how you feel about yourself, and the words you use to affirm and describe who you are. Dr. Grant is a firm believer that true beauty starts from the inside then it comes out. Explains Dr. Grant on the subject of inner beauty:

It's what I do on the inner plane that maintains what I do on the outer plane, it's what I think inside my head that makes me look like I do. I am in love with Gwendolyn. I look into the mirror and I talk all kinds of romantic talk to myself-I'm never going to put Gwendolyn down! So when I look into that mirror, I give Gwendolyn all of the talk necessary to nurture herself, because I don't have the right to abuse myself verbally!

Did you catch that last verse? You *"Don't have the right to abuse [yourself] verbally!"* Quick translation: God don't like ugly, because God don't make ugly-especially you! To affirm otherwise is blasphemy!

How To Write Your Own Affirmations

The technique of writing self-empowering affirmations is to always write them in the "now" moment- as if you were already in possession of the very thing that you are affirming. Never speak an affirmation in the past or future tense. For example:

"I would like to love myself more,"

or

"I will love myself more."

These type of affirmations, puts the manifestation of your desires in the past or future tense. These are the kinds of affirmations that keep your desires unfulfilled and never in the present moment. Right NOW is the only moment in time that you will ever experience ANYTHING, so why put your desires and dreams behind you or in front of you?

It is most unfortunate, but most of the dialogue we use on our behalf leans toward the negative rather than the positive. Negative self-talk keeps you from being able to accept a compliment, from feeling worthy or deserving of affirming your attractiveness, and it keeps you from feeling good about yourself-lowering your self-value, worth and esteem.

Experts say we talk to ourselves on average about 400 to 600 words per minute, but most of the words we speak compounds preordained stresses, anxieties and unhappiness. It's also true that the words we use to describe ourselves and how we feel is very limited. Linguists say that an average person's working vocabulary consists of only between 2,000 and 10,000 words. With a conservative estimate, the English language contains half a million words, which means we regularly use only 1/2 of 1% to 2% of the entire English language!

So to create a Positive Self-Image, you must learn how to focus on using positive words to describe yourself and your emotions, since there are more negative words to describe your emotions than there are positive ones, discipline is a must. There are about 1,051 words to describe positive emotions in the English language, but there are about 2,086 words to describe negative emotions. So make a covenant with yourself and make a conscious, deliberate effort to elect words that will empower your moods and emotions. Ok? Thank you.

Here are ten PSI affirmations that I have used on myself and others with great consequences. They will help you raise your esteem, while in your morning. I also suggest that you try and create your own affirmations to describe exactly what you want, and affirm your personal needs.

SPECIAL QUICK TIP:Affirmations to use

Use these affirmations while looking in the mirror and speak your name where the blanks appear in the affirmation.

1) YOU ARE MY MOST PRIZED POSSESSION _____. I LOVE YOU, I CHERISH YOU AND I ADORE YOU!

2) I LOVE AND APPRECIATE YOU _____ JUST THE WAY YOU ARE, EACH DAY YOU IMPROVE MORE AND MORE!

3) YOU ARE ONE OF THE MOST BEAUTIFUL PERSONS I'VE EVER SEEN _____, YOU LOOK GOOD, YOU FEEL GOOD BECAUSE YOU ARE GOOD-GOOD AT EVERYTHING YOU DO!

4) I AM NOW BALANCED IN MY WORK, I AM NOW BALANCED IN MY HEALTH, I AM NOW BALANCED IN MY RELATIONSHIPS, I AM NOW BALANCED IN MY EMOTIONS AND ALL AREAS OF MY LIFE. I WILL LET NOTHING MAKE ME LOSE SIGHT OF THIS REALITY!

5) YOU ARE ENERGY IN EXPRESSION _____, AND YOU HAVE LOTS OF IT!

6) YOU ARE VIBRANTLY HEALTHY AND RADIANTLY BEAUTIFUL _____ RIGHT NOW AND ALWAYS! NOTHING AND NO ONE CAN MAKE YOU FEEL UNATTRACTIVE!

7) ALL THINGS ARE NOW WORKING TOGETHER FOR THE GOOD IN MY LIFE. I DESERVE THE BEST BECAUSE I AM THE BEST.

8) EVERYTHING YOU COULD EVER WANT _____, YOU ALREADY HAVE. I CLAIM IT AND I ACCEPT IT RIGHT NOW!

9) I AM RELAXED AND CENTERED. AND I HAVE TIME FOR EVERYTHING THAT I WANT TO DO.

10) THIS IS MY DAY. THIS IS MY WAY. I HAVE FOCUS AND I HAVE FAITH. THE WORLD IS MINE!

PART 4

THE MORNING MOTIVE

Defining The Theme Of Your Look

Now that we have your attitude in check, it's now time to establish the motive or theme of your new self-image. The theme of your makeup should reflect your mood and what you plan to accomplish for the day. Personality and individual taste should be the two main ingredients when defining the motive of your image. The colors in your wardrobe selection should also play a significant role in your choice of cosmetic colors.

Your look should be easy on the eye and very simple to apply; never wearing wardrobe colors that fight for attention with your eye, cheek and lip color. Harmony of hue and color compliment is forever the rule of thumb. For instance, if you're wearing a red dress, you wouldn't use orange or pinkish shades to brighten your face would you? No! Instead you'd use browns on the eyes and neutral browns or reds on the lip.

Another rule of thumb is trying not to have your face fighting for attention. In other words, if you're going to use a vibrant lip color like a red, orange or pink, then you should tone down the colors you use on your eyes. Conversely, if you're really going to play up your eyes, then go gentle on the intensity of the lip shade.

Visualizing Your Motive

One technique that can be used to help you define your look for the day is simply to visualize the night before what attire you're going to wear and the cosmetic colors you want to use, then imagine how you'd like to look and feel while wearing them. Not only are women turning toward visualization to relieve stress and meditative self-help, but there are a great deal of women using the technique to accommodate all sorts of events and personal activities in their life, planning and projecting a Positive Self-Image is just one of them.

Beauty is always based on where your attention is focused. If your mood and attention is upbeat with high expectations, then the colors you'll choose, more than likely, in both wardrobe and makeup will be powerful and commanding to compliment those emotions. Conversely, if your personality tends to be depressed with angst and threatened self-esteem, your color selection may very well be drab and lifeless. In this case, it really won't matter what brand of cosmetics you use or how well you apply them, the outcome will be less than desirable, because your mood and attitude is less than desirable.

Remember, cosmetics is an attitude to be worn, not something you wear to have an attitude. Shine on the inside more and never attempt to follow trends designed by and for other people. If you become a master of your own self-image and set your own style, trends and image scripture then you'll become a walking beauty book that other women will want to read and follow!

To help you visualize and focus your attention on the theme you wish to represent for the day, fill out the list of questions below.

- WHAT AM I HAPPY ABOUT WITH MY SELF-IMAGE RIGHT NOW?

- WHAT AM I ENJOYING MOST WITH MY SELF-IMAGE RIGHT NOW?

- WHAT AM I GRATEFUL ABOUT WITH MY SELF-IMAGE RIGHT NOW?

- WHAT WOULD I LIKE TO IMPROVE WITH MY SELF-IMAGE RIGHT NOW?

- WHAT COLORS COME TO MY MIND WHEN I THINK HAPPY THOUGHTS?

- WHAT FASHION AND MAKEUP COMBINATION MAKE ME LOOK FABULOUS!

Remember, self-assessment always leads to self-fulfillment. Just before retiring for the evening, find a quiet spot in the house and take a look at this exercise and use the visualization techniques that you've learned and notice how easy your image motive will come to you upon awakening in the morning.

15 Relaxation Techniques To End A Stressful Day

There is nothing more important to your inner and outer health and beauty than learning how to relax. In learning how to properly relax and release your inner frustrations you will get an extra boost in the morning, helping you to better achieve your goals for the day.

Here are 15 relaxation activities that you can use in conjunction with all of the techniques you have already learned. Make a special attempt to relax before and/or after meditation and ascribe to actress Karyn Parsons philosophy and find things that make you happy. She says, "Surround yourself with the things that you like and the people you like, and do what you like. Some of us have trouble being selfish. You have to make yourself selfish once in a while-take care of yourself and make sure you are happy."

1. YELLING A COMMAND: STOP, CANCEL or FREEZE!

When you find yourself unable to focus or concentrate on anything other than daily problems and challenges, in your mind or if you're somewhere where there's no people, yell as loud as you can STOP, CANCEL or FREEZE; then immediately repeat to yourself one of the aforementioned affirmations.

2. WATER RELAXATION:

You were carried for nine months in water, and you loved to play in it when you were a baby. Water is the most soothing physical elixir. Immersing oneself in a hot, soothing

bath should be implemented daily. Bathing, steaming, or whirlpooling will relax even the most stressed.

3. EXERCISE:

Believe it or not, but a good workout can greatly relax you. A light aerobic workout, a couple of laps around the pool, or jogging a mile or two can set the tone for relaxation and getting away from it all.

4. Seeing the fruits of your exercise labor can RAISE SELF-ESTEEM and improve your body-image.

Bertice Berry says the memory of her once weighing over 250 pounds still hovers in her mind. To negate the old vision of herself, she says, *"I work out 5:00 every morning. I have a trainer who comes over and we do some form of weight lifting and speed walking."*

5. MUSCLE RELAXATION:

Sit quietly in a room and tense and contract your muscles, then release them as you breathe, or practice different forms of Yoga. Former Entertainment Tonight reporter, Lisa Canning says Yoga is her mind/body elixir. *"I do it only a few times a week, and it really helps me to relax."* Yoga is a sure fire way to remove tension in muscles from the strain of a hectic day. Also try facial exercises and self-massage used in conjunction with water relaxation for a total mind/body, tension release.

6. STRETCHING AND BREATHING:

During a full day of work, your muscles can become tense and restricted. By using breathing and stretching techniques, you'll loosen up your body, and desensitize the day that's passed. Five minutes a day of stretching and breathing can really stretch your endurance for the day and the next.

7. AROMATHERAPY:

Surrounding yourself with your favorite scents and fragrances is an automatic relaxing agent. The scent of vanilla has been proven to be one of the most soothing aromas on the market. Aromacologists say it reminds us of vanilla ice cream when we were kids.

Philippe Matthews

8. LISTENING TO MUSIC:

Jazz, classical, new age and light rock are the sounds of choice. Come home, make a cup of herbal tea, put the headphones on and take a trip. You deserve it. Don't feel guilty, don't think about work, just merely exist!

9. NATURE WALKING:

Taking a quiet walk in a neighboring park, forest or woods is a wonderful way to press away from the daily onslaughts of the world. It is also a good form of exercise, and creates peace of mind. Try walking for 15 to 30 minutes every other day, and watch your stress disappear.

10. READING:

Poetry, the bible, personal empowerment literature, anything that will uplift you should be read to keep your awareness on your Light. Reading is a naturally wonderful way to maintain your focus and discipline of peace and harmony.

11. ENGAGING IN MINDLESS ENTERTAINMENT:

Sometimes you just don't want to think about anything,! So when this happens, don't fight it, let it have its way with you. Be a couch potato and watch Dave's Stupid Human Tricks! There's nothing wrong with a little escapism now and then!

12. DAYDREAMING:

Let your mind wander far away. Just let it drift. Sometimes, you'll be amazed how relaxing this is. Remember, daydreaming is not controlled mental imaging, its random thinking, so paint pretty pictures in your mind that will add to your relaxation.

13. LAUGHING FOR COMIC RELIEF:

Laughter is good for the soul. Find something, anything to get tickled about. Former talk show hostess, Rolonda Watts in an interview gave me the secret to her happiness. *"I laugh a lot!"* she said. *"That's what keeps me happy and shining. I love to laugh and I believe that makes you live longer, it keeps you well. I'm very fulfilled, and it doesn't get better than this."*

14. SPENDING TIME WITH LOVED ONES:

Family and friends are sometimes a good escape if you're close, and they pose no added stress. Communion with others can often times be the very thing we need to shake away the blues, relax and enjoy the moment.

Pop diva Karyn White says she loves spending time with people who are beautiful on the inside. *"Most of my friends have to have that quality. I love fun people, honest people, giving people-I hate negative people. A beautiful person, a beautiful spirit-that's beauty to me."*

15. COMPANIONSHIP:

Spending time caring for a cat, dog, plant or goldfish can in its own way add to your relaxation. Pets and hobbies are another quality blues buster to relieving stress.

16. MAKING LOVE:

Researchers surveyed fifty-one women who suffered frequent migraines and found that twenty-four of them reported improvement or full recovery when they had sexual relations. It seems that during orgasm the body releases endorphins-the body's own natural painkillers-they play a significant role in reducing headache pain. It is reported that in less than 1% of people, orgasm can actually cause a headache. Sorry, the old *"I got a headache honey"* routine won't cut it anymore. So share life with your soul mate, hug and snug, and make all the negatives of the day go away. Always find time to love the one that loves you.

What Nine Divas Do To Relax

It's part of every entertainer's job to look great -- on screen or on stage. These ten divas know that a truly healthy glow can only come from a balanced lifestyle -- with plenty of time for rest and relaxation. Here's how the stars get their "R & R."

Cree Summer, television actress

What does she do to get away from it all? *"I'm always away from it all!"* she says, *"I write songs, I sing, I write poetry and read it aloud. I also like animals and babies -- I'd like to have lots and lots of babies!"* Cree has a love for the mountains, as well as the valley breezes when she's cruising on her 1969 Morgan Speedster Roughrider or her renegade Harley Davidson.

Lisa Fischer, Grammy Award winner, R&B singer

Whether she is singing one of her own soulful songs, or reminiscing about crooning in the background for Luther Vandross, Lisa Fischer is a dynamo of fashion and entertainment. But, off-stage, Lisa says, *"I'm very relaxed. I like jeans, my little black leggings, big sweaters and boots. I don't wear any makeup during the day. I can walk down the street and no one recognizes me, which is wonderful."*

Karyn Parsons, television and movie actress

Quiet time is almost non-existent for Karyn, but she finds refreshment among close friends. *"I'm lucky. I have a lot of good friends around me that have always been there for me. They've known me forever, so I like just hanging' out with them more than anything else... I don't have a retreat."* Karyn is actively involved with charities, especially those relating to children and world hunger. *"Anything that comes along having to do with children, I'll say 'yes' to!"* she explains. *"One of my big things is feeding people and kids."*

Ann Bennett-Nesby, lead singer of Sounds of Blackness

If Ann isn't on stage or in the studio singing, you'll probably find her at home, listening to her musical favorites -- Aretha Franklin, Patti Labelle, Ella Fitzgerald, Donny Hathaway and Luther Vandross. She says she also loves to read and go to church.

Dawnn Lewis, actress, singer, songwriter

"Children are important to me because I'm one of the biggest kids I know," says Dawnn. *"Sometimes I think I'm a dreamer and optimist to a fault. I still believe in my dream, and I'm going to keep believing in my dream."* Dawnn finds meaning in motivating children to follow their own stars, in her work with UNICEF, the

National 4-H Foundation, United Negro College Fund, the Office of Substance Abuse Prevention, the Camp Fire Boys and Girls Club, and Planned Parenthood. Dawnn explains, *"I think too many young people today don't have a dream. They have let their reality squelch any hope of having a dream and the reality of their existence is stronger than what their dreams could ever be"*.

"I believe as much as I've been blessed, and as much as I've been granted in my lifetime, that I need to encourage as many kids as I can to believe in their dreams. The only reason I'm where I am is because I stuck to the hope of my dreams possibly coming true."

Tina Lifford, actress, screenwriter

Tina Lifford sees relaxation as living in a state of universal harmony, and balancing one's energies. She says, *"One of the most important things is that by lessening the 'alien' within, you increase. The aliens come in many, many shapes and forms, and most of those shapes and forms are boxes that society and we ourselves have placed ourselves in. It's my intention to live in this world without the boxes, and the limitations that have been accepted by the mass consciousness of the human race. It is our job to kill the alien within."*

Mavis Staples, vocal and musical legend

Mavis Staples' relaxation comes from giving to others, and offering a message that positively affects people's lives. She says, *"I like to give a message that can help somebody and lift somebody. People need to hear something that will lift them up."*

Patrice Rushen, musician, singer, songwriter

Patrice believes that the most important step to learning how to relax is gaining peace of mind. *"I want to be able to sleep at night, so I try to live a little each day and do things that allow me to feel good about myself. And when you feel good about yourself, I think somehow you begin to give that off in everything."*

Yolanda Adams, gospel singer

More than anything in the world, Yolanda loves spending time with her family. She says, *"I could not do anything without my family. I'm a very outgoing, witty person, but when I'm at home, I only want my family around, because I know they're sincere, and I know they mean the best for me. I keep my family real close to me, and I don't let a lot of people in. I'm very private."*

SPECIAL QUICK TIP:Aromatherapy and Relaxation

The science of scent is known as aromatherapy or aromachology,. The effect of scent in tandem with meditation, visualization or any of the 15 relaxation techniques can greatly expand your sense of self-awareness. The power of scent is a worldwide phenomenon. At wealthy Hindu weddings, it's customary to erect a silk canopy over the bride and groom, while burning beneath it is a sacred fire of fragrant sandalwood and aromatic gums. During the ceremony these aromatic essences fill the tent with savory fumes. The use of fragrant baths to protect and purify the body is also very common in Brazil, particularly in the region of the Amazon and among the population of African descent.

How You Smell

The science of scent is as spectacular as it is sensory. The Olfactory Research Fund says an odor has its origins first as an aroma molecule. Normal perception of odors, fragrance and aromas would not be possible if these molecules did not first enter our nose. When we sniff, currents of air swirl up through our nostrils, over the bony turbinate, to a small "sheet" about the size of a postage stamp, which contains millions of receptor cells. This is called the olfactory epithelium.

Each of the millions of sensory (receptor) cells has minuscule filaments or cilia extending from protrusions of the cell-olfactory knobs, located at the tip of an elongation of the nerve. The cilia contain proteins that grasp for aroma molecules-not every cilia interacts with the molecules-however, if the appropriate aroma molecule and receptor fuse, a sequence of events is initiated. The sensory cell is excited, electrical activity rushes from within and ultimately the perception of an odor emerges.

SPECIAL QUICK TIP: The sound of music

Remember, Susan Taylor's morning regime? She begins her day at 5:30 in the morning with a hot bath, laced with fragrant oils, surrounded by scented candles while listening to a meditation tape.

There are many kind of meditation tapes to choose from in the marketplace, however, one series that I use in my training classes, and found to have the most impact of relieving stress and countermanding stress before it even occurs is the music of Maharishi Gandharva-Ved. Gandharva-Ved's music is produced by Maharishi Ayur-Ved and steeped in Indian philosophy and tradition with noted followers such as Deepak Chopra.

Maharishi Gandharva-Ved is said to be the eternal music of nature, the classic music of the ancient Vedic civilization which enjoyed heaven on earth. Thousands of years ago, its musical formulas were created by the Vedic sages to perfectly match nature's own rhythms and cycles. The purpose is to neutralize stress in the environment and create a harmonizing balance for those who listen to its soothing flute music.

Their philosophy also purports that there are different rhythms and frequencies throughout nature, and throughout every level of creation. One frequency melds into the other and the process of change occurs. At the dawn of a new day, there is a special quality of freshness in the atmosphere, at noon there is a like quality, and in the evening there is yet another.

The ancient Gandharva-Ved sages understood these natural frequencies so well that they created specific musical compositions, or ragas, to mirror the natural changing rhythms that succeed at different times of the day and night.

According to this philosophy, the 24-hour clock is divided into eight Gandharva-Ved time periods, each of which is three hours in length. Gandharva-Ved music has a system that covers all the day and night time periods. So you would choose one of their one hour tapes, and listen according to the time of day that is most convenient to relieve stress. For example, if you wanted to begin your day getting in tune with flute harmonies of nature, you'd choose the ragas for 4-7 a.m. Likewise, if you wanted to calm the end of your day and soothe yourself to sleep, you'd listen to the Evening tape from 7-10 p.m.

Gandharva-Ved music can be used as background music, to relax your regular activities, during meditation, or, if your schedule will permit, just lying around the house, listening with your eyes closed.

The 8 Gandharva-Ved Time Periods

- Early Morning: 4am-7am Morning: 7am-10-am Midday: 10am-1pm Afternoon: 1pm-4pm

- Early Evening: 4pm-7pm Evening: 7pm-10-pm Midnight: 10pm-1am Late Night: 1am-4am

- Gandharva-Ved music is available on both CD and tape formats. For information of how to order these tapes, or for a brochure call (800) 255-8332.

PART 5

IN THE MIRROR

SKIN CARE FOR WOMEN ON THE MOVE

The most important aspect to beautiful skin is using high-quality skin care products and developing a good skincare regimen. Good skin offers you a good canvas for the story of cosmetic color to be told. Image icon Iman believes that good skin care represents beauty from the inside out. She says, *"Many women have become too dependent on color systems. If you can't walk out of the house without makeup and feel great about your skin, you have problems."* She also believes that education is a key ingredient to healthy skin. *"We have to start by dispelling the myths-we're not made of steel. Sunlight, pollution and stress affect our skin, too. Looking your best means having the best skin possible. Many women use makeup as a mask to hide behind and forget to take care of their skin."*

WATER: That Essential Skin Care Ingredient

Before we get involved with skin care treatments, I'd like to take a moment and introduce you to on one of the most important ingredients in skin care products-water! H20 consumes about 75% of the earth and 65% of our bodies-greatly affecting the appearance of our skin. Water is also the most abundant of all substances and is the most vital of all nutrients to human existence, parallel with the air we breathe.

Everyday scientists discover new applications from the seas such as, plankton, seaweed's, and shellfish. All of these elements contain an abundance of natural components that are essential to life. Mineral salts like calcium, potassium, sodium, silica, and magnesium are also present in water as well as elements such as iodine, glucides, mucilages, amino-acids, and vitamins A, B, C, D E, and chlorophyll. These components are essential for bodily functions, growth, tissue regeneration, reinforcing organic defenses, constitution and maintenance of our bone structure, and metabolic regulation.

Some scientists purport that in the beginning of evolution, everything came from the sea; some 3.8 billion years ago, it was from the waters of the oceans and seas that the first forms of vegetal and animal life sprang. The healthy influence of water in our bodies is evident in people who have a radiant, glowing complexion with minimal blemishes, if any at all. A substantial intake of water is mandatory for a healthy face and body-image, especially if you are the type of women who is constantly in flight and jumping from climate to climate. This kind of lifestyle can cause major dehydration.

The Culprits Of Dehydration

There are several things that can cause skin dehydration: excessive exercise, low water intake, and extended exposure to the sun are just a few, but it is plane travel that ranks numero uno. Cindy Herron of the musical group En Vogue says, *"When you fly long distances for some reason flying dehydrates you. My mother told me that flight attendant's skin ages faster because they fly all of the time and it's such a dry atmosphere, so you should have a moisturizer for the skin and drink a lot of water. I read for every hour that you fly, you need to drink eight ounces of water."*

The nurturing effects of water was also very important to soul singer Vesta when she was done performing after a show. She told me, *"The first thing I want is an ice cold glass of water. When I come off the stage, I'm so dehydrated, because I work so hard I perspire."* Vesta's water necessity doesn't end when she comes off stage from performing either, she shared the same position at home as well. *"To relax at home,"* she says, *"I like to take a nice hot shower. I have a really great shower in my house and you can sit down in the shower and just let the water bead on you."*

To keep your skin healthy and hydrated, drink at least six 8-ounce glasses of mineral-rich water daily. You can use tap "hard" water if it's high in mineral content. You can call your local water department and ask them for the number of grains of calcium and magnesium per gallon of H_2O. 4 to 10 grains per gallon is considered hard water, and 11 to 19 grains is considered extra hard water.

But if your water is soft with less than 4 grains per gallon, or if your tap water is just plain tasteless, you can stock up on bottled mineral waters. Evian water or Vittel are tasty Still waters from France. Vichy Celestine and Perrier are French bubblies. Another Still water imported from Italy is Fiuggi, and a good bubbly is San Pellegrino also from Italy.

A Word About Body Care

Water plays a significant role in the appearance of your total body skin. Whether it's cleansing products or moisturizing products, water is also an essential ingredient in your body care treatments. Singer/songwriter Cherrelle told me she was very much into body creams. *"Body creams are very important in my life, I can't live without them."*

She uses Tiffany body oils in her bath water and also likes the fragrant both oils of Carolina Herrera, and Paris by Yves Saint Laurent. Cherrelle is a bath gel and body cream connoisseur and says there's nothing like a great water escape. *"I try to use the same body cream as the bath gel...oh what a feeling!"*

Model turned actress and television commentator Lisa Canning ascribes to a unique, yet very efficient method of moisturizing her body. She says, *"I use a body scrub and a loofah everyday. And I use honey all over my skin when I go into the sauna...it's a great moisturizer for the skin."* Using the heat from the sauna, your own body moisture begins to work in alchemy with the honey (a natural moisturizer), putting you in a sticky situation, but effective nonetheless.

Companies With Good Body Care Systems

Arden's Spa Collection is defined by four moods: Tranquility, Sensual, Euphorics, and Exhilarators, each with its own mood-enhancing color and aromatic fragrance notes. For example, Tranquilities (meaning water) is represented by the color Aquamarine with fragrances of the sea, setting the mood for relaxation, de-stressing and deep calming.

Elizabeth Arden is now in association with Compagnie Fermiere des Eaux et des Bains de Spa of Belgium, a company that is the leading exporter of bottled waters in Europe. The two companies have agreed to form a unique venture, which is the inclusion of Spa Natural Spring Water into selected Arden products.

The partnership is to celebrate the virtual essence of all health: water. The Belgian Spa baths have been enthusiastically sought for their medicinal properties since the first century A.D. The Spa Thermal Establishment has been for centuries a symbol of the spring waters-the purest and most famous in Europe. They also inspired Elizabeth Arden's Maine Chance Spa, the first true beauty spa in America that was founded on many of the same age-old principles of total well being.

Anti-Aging Waters

Water also plays an integral role in anti-aging skin care products as the natural course of age and photo-damaging breeds fine lines and wrinkles to appear on the face and around the eyes. From the Italy based spa Terme di Montecatini, Princess Marcella Borghese's Concentrato di Vita is a targeted treatment containing the highest concentration of their Aqua di Vita, meaning "Living Water." This special non-oily formula hydrates areas of your face that are particularly prone to fine lines and comes in a pack of six serum vials that are to be used day and night to immediately help restore youth and elasticity to your skin-perfect for travel!

Borghese's Living Water can also be found in their Fango Active Mud for Face and Body. I've personally recommended this famous mud treatment of Montecatini for years. It gives over-stressed skin a new surge of vitality, releasing moisture deep into the epidermal skin layer while the nutrients in the volcanic mud work to remove embedded impurities, push water deep into the skin, and causes skin to have an overall radiance. Fango Active Mud should be used at least once a week in conjunction with your regular body/face care routine. You should also know that Borghese's products are also devoid of any known irritants and fragrances, making great for sensitive skin's.

QUICK TIP:

If you're traveling and forgot to bring your shower gel, dilute 1 part of scented shampoo like The Body Shop's Orange Spice Shampoo to 6 parts of water, lather up and shower away!

QUICK TIP:

Note that soaking or showering in very hot water is not good for your skin's overall appearance. Extreme heat can dry your skin, because moisture will be lost much faster as your body begins to cool down. Warm water is the absolute best, allowing you to stay in and soak for about 20 minutes without any damage. The ideal water temperature for your bath is about 95'F. In fact, if the water is too hot, it will even tire you out, and the heat may encourage tiny spider veins to appear on your legs.

SPECIAL QUICK TIP: Water And Preservatives

Beauty products that don't contain water last almost forever. Diametrically, the higher the content of water is within a product the sooner the product will spoil, and bacteria loves to breed in water as opposed to other more exotic ingredients. Oil-based and glycerin based products have a much longer shelf life than those that do not.

A natural biocidal (bacteria killing) preservative is glycerin. With high longevity, glycerin destroys bacteria and is usually great for women with problem skin. Cosmetics that contain alcohol also have a longer life, because alcohol is one of the best germ killers. However, the down side of some alcohol based products is that it can have a drying effect on the skin. Beauty products that house preservatives should last up to two years with the exception of eye makeup. Also, any beauty products that you have at home, or are homemade, should be kept in the refrigerator, because the cold is a natural curb of germ growth.

Some popular names used to describe preservatives are words like methylparaben, propylparaben, butylparaben, potassium sorbate, quaternium-15, and dehydroacetic acid. Products with paraben are purported to be the best preservatives because they're derived from benzoic acid, a natural substance chemically treated to fight bacteria. Look on the back of labels for the names of some of these preservatives.

QUICK TIP:

Has this ever happened to you? You packed your beauty kit, arrived at your destination only to find out that your creams and toners jostled open because of the natural turbulence of planes, trains or automobiles? Well to make sure this doesn't happen to you again, seal your jars and bottles securely by melting together equal amounts of candle wax and petroleum jelly, then brush the mixture around the cap and neck of the jars and bottles and let dry naturally.

SPECIAL QUICK TIP:The skin care of sun care

Since 70 percent of your lifetime to sun exposure occurred during your childhood, it only makes sense to protect your skin from the sun's ultraviolet rays as your timeline continues to pass on.

Sunscreens reflect and absorb damaging UVA rays that penetrate your skin, causing sunburn and at its extreme skin cancer. The most common reflective ingredient in sunscreens is titanium dioxide (the active ingredient in most "chemical-free" sunscreens).

UV reduces your skin's immune defenses, marring your complexion and creating skin coarseness. UV also makes your skin sag and lose its elasticity and the more sun you're exposed to, the sooner photoaging occurs. Both UVA and UVB rays damage your skin's DNA at the epidermal (outer) layer. For this very reason, a quality sunscreen is highly recommended.

It is never too early to develop early sun care habits. In fact, it should be considered essential for quality skin and is evident in many tests. One test conducted by the National Skin Cancer

Awareness Committee studied 588 Australians, (Australians have the highest skin cancer rate anywhere in the world). It is said that two out of three Australians develop skin cancer at some point in their life. Having 1 to 30 solar keratoses (red, flaky lesions on their skin), considered such factors for non-melanoma skin cancer. Half the subjects were given an SPF (Sun Protection Factor) of 17 to be used daily, while the other half got a lotion with no active ingredient. At the end of the seven month study, the sunscreen group had 35 percent fewer new lesions and 8 percent more remissions.

In another study, a group of epidemiologist's came to the conclusion that using sunscreen for the first eighteen years of your life would reduce the likelihood of producing non-melanoma skin cancer by about 78 percent. This skin trivia has caused dermatologists to create a new ingredient in today's sunscreens and self-tanners called Dihydroxyacetone (DHA). Its a colorless, powder or liquid molecule similar to sugar. DHA received FDA approval as a food colorant years ago, and when applied to your skin's outer layer, it mixes with your skin's natural proteins and creates a brownish color. The artificial tan that DHA produces lasts about three to five days on the skin, until your skin naturally exfoliates.

The average self-tanner takes about 30 to 45 minutes to dry on the skin, but some newer brands like Clinique's Self-Tan Spray Mist for the Body dries in 10 minutes. Doctor's have also developed a unique delivery system for these self-tanners such as water-in-silicone emulsions that spread the product evenly for quicker and more uniformed tanning development and drying. Self-tanners containing DHA are not considered sunscreens, in order for them to protect your skin from the sun they have to have an SPF as well. Princess Marcella Borghese's Solare Superiore Sun Care SPF 15 or Erno Lazlo's Self Tanning Lotion SPF 8 are quality examples. Then there's Bain de Soleil's SPF + Color Sunscreen and Self-Tanner with an impressive SPF of 30 for maximum protection.

You should know that sunscreens are only meant to sit on top of your skin's surface to have any impact on blocking out harmful rays. When you rub the sunscreen into your skin, you reduce its effectiveness. According to research, rubbing an SPF 15 into your skin turns into an SPF 12 by the time absorption occurs. You should also know that reapplying your sunscreen throughout the day will not offer you any extra sun protection. If you use a sunscreen that allows you to stay in the sun for an hour and a half, then that's all the time you have, regardless of how many times you reapply the product. In other words, an SPF of 8 equals SPF 8 -- not SPF 16. Only reapply your sunscreen if you've been sweating heavily and have toweled most of it off. And be liberal when applying your sunscreen.

Aside from using moderate quantities of sunscreen lotion, you should know that your clothing can also add extra protection for deflecting ultraviolet rays. An average cotton T-shirt blocks out 90 percent of the suns rays with an SPF of 10, and 94 percent with an SPF of 15. Wearing a hat is another good amendment to your sunscreen protection. A four-inch brimmed hat will cut down on the radiation on your face and neck by about 70 percent.

If you have money to spare, you can spend up to $50 for a basic T-shirt, along with other SPF clothing. That's right! Garments designed to protect your skin from the suns rays. The FDA considers these garments medical devices because they are sunscreens. Sun Precautions is a Seattle-based company who's Solumbra line includes jackets, T-shirts and nylon pants with a SPF of 30. Nylon is a tightly woven fabric that is said to be more sun protection friendly than many other fabrics. In Arizona, FrogSkin, Inc claims its nylon clothing protects with an Sun Protection Factor of 36 and Chicago's Solar Protective Factory purports their hats and nylon garments block out up to 99 percent of the suns damaging rays.

Where Can You Burn?

- Under an umbrella (sand reflects 20 percent of UV rays)

- On the water (calm water reflects 3 percent of UV)

- In the water (75 percent of UV penetrates to 30 feet)

- Up on the slopes (snow reflects 85 percent of UV)

- In the city (concrete kicks back 45 percent of UV)

- Through your clothes (a cotton tee lets in up to 60 percent of UV)

- In the park (grass reflects 3 percent of UV)

SKIN CARE 101: The Basic Three Of Beauty

There are literally thousands of skin care products on the market to choose from, and even more directions on how to use them. But the KIS principle of Keeping It Simple is highly recommended when producing your own skin care regimen. Stripping your skin system down to the bare bones is just what Karyn Parsons learned from one of the Makeup Artist on The Fresh Prince Of Bel Air:

I've tried so many things. I would buy the most expensive products to have wonderful skin. Because I was real lucky in high school, I didn't break out very much. It wasn't until I got out of high school that I started breaking out. [On the show] my skin kept getting really weird, it was bumpy or it would break out and I was trying all of this stuff. [The makeup artist on the show] said, 'Why don't you just stop using everything and go back to whatever you could think of when your skin was ok-back to something really basic?' I went back to using Ivory soap and Oil Of Olay moisturizer-stuff that I can buy at a drugstore. And my skin cleared up.

Even Rolonda Watts admits she doesn't have any strict beauty routine. Instead she uses Clarins and Kheil's skin care products and makes sure she cleanses her skin at least twice daily to remove all traces of makeup from the day.

So become brilliant at the skin care basics when choosing what I call the Three Basic routine. The Three Basic consists of a cleanser, a toner, and a moisturizer. This is your foundational skin care system. Facials, mud masks and other products outside of this three step process is considered specialty or maintenance care.

Pop singer, Karyn White says she gets *"facials every week and I try not to wear a lot of makeup. When I don't have to, I wear just powder on my face. I make sure that I wash my face with Shiseido Revitalizing Cleanser, also their Revitalizing Cream,"* for moisture protection. Karyn also remembers the importance of water as she makes a point to eat right and drink plenty of water to flush her skin and system of impurities.

Steps To A Three Basic Skin Care System

STEP ONE: Cleansing

Skin cleansers come in liquid, lotion, creme, and bar soap form. It is the most important treatment you can give your skin. Its sole purpose is to remove makeup, dirt, oil and debris from your skin. Some women prefer to use cleansing lotions or creams, (some of which are used without water, while others can be rinsed off if desired.) Many women, however, prefer soap and water.

As long as a gentle complexion soap or beauty bar is used, soap and water does no harm to the skin. In fact, it cleanses skin more thoroughly than many of the lotions or creams on the market. But try not to cleanse your skin no more than twice a day as not to strip your skin of natural moisture.

APPLICATION: Cleanser

a) Apply cleanser to the five facial motor points: nose, chin, forehead and both cheeks, avoiding the eye area completely.

b) Use upward and outward motions on your face, paying careful attention around the eye area, because tissue is delicate.

c) Splash face with water at least seven times to completely rinse away surface cleanser.

QUICK TIP:

Never use a colored wash cloth on your face. Over a course of time, the dyes in a colored washcloth becomes embedded in your skin's epidermal layer, and can cause discoloration. Always use a clean, white wash cloth.

QUICK TIP:

I bet you didn't know that a natural deep pore cleanser is milk of magnesia. To cleanse your skin, take a couple of dollops and spread on your face with a cotton ball. Avoid your eye area and leave milk of magnesia on for about 10 minutes then remove with a warm (white) washcloth and apply your moisturizer as usual.

STEP TWO: Toning

Toners, fresheners, clarifiers and astringents are all basically the same product, except they vary in oil absorbing properties and alcohol percentage. Toners are used to remove excess cleanser and oils from your skin and to tighten your pores and bring the skin back to its normal PH (acid) balance. Toners can also be viewed as a second cleanser, although optional as many dermatologists say that toning is not necessarily a needed procedure in cleansing the skin. It does, however, add to the freshness and overall glow of the skin.

APPLICATION: Toner

a)   Using a cotton ball, sweep toner over your entire face, avoiding the eye area.

b)   You should not see any residue left on the cotton ball after using the toner, if so, repeat the process until skin is thoroughly cleansed.

QUICK TIP:

Traveling from climate to climate can cause overnight breakouts or blackhead eruptions to occur on your skin. A wonderful travel remedy that you can try is adding a small amount of alum (found in drugstores) to 2 ounces of witch hazel. Shake well and apply it to your skin's blemish and allow to dry. Leave the serum on all day, with or without makeup.

STEP THREE: Moisturizing

A moisturizers main purpose is to help seal in the natural moisture mantle of your skin. Moisturizers come in basically two formulations; lotions and creams. Oily skin needs less help with moisturizer since its oil content provides a natural moisture seal, but oily skin still needs moisture.

APPLICATION: Moisturizer

  a) Moisturizer should be applied morning and night if your skin has tendencies toward dryness.

  b) It is absolutely vital to use gentle upward movements when applying moisturizer on your face.

  c) Use only a dollop of moisturizer, because the heavier the cream, the less you should use-the weight of the cream could damage skin.

  d) Apply moisturizer to your forehead, nose, chin and both cheeks.

  e) Massage the lotion or cream in quickly and lightly, beginning at your chin and moving up across the cheeks to the ears, then down and around the nose, and up from the nose to the temples, then across the forehead. Treat the eye area even more gently.

  f) Don't forget to moisturize your neck and throat as well, using long strokes from your collarbone to your jaw.

QUICK TIP:

Apply moisturizer to your dampened face, then take a fluffy, dry face towel and put your blow-dryer near it until the towel gets warm. Apply it to your face and it will help seal in the water plus your moisturizer. Caution: Don't use the blow-dryer in or near a water-filled tub, or when you're wet.

SPECIAL QUICK TIP: The ABC's of AHA's

If you're a woman on the go, you well know that the buzz word in skin care for the mom in motion is been AHA's, an acronym for Alpha Hydroxy Acids. This ingredient has permeated almost every beauty product, from foot and face creams to nail and body lotions. The purpose behind this ingredient is they offer women something very important and necessary-faster skin cell renewal and decreased appearance of aging!

As you age, skin cell renewal wanes and may slowly break down the youthful appearance of your skin. If you lead an active lifestyle, loaded with hectic scheduling, then you literally speed up the slowing down of your skin's youthful appearance.

Dr. Cheryl Burgess, dermatologist and creator of the Black Opal skin care system, distributed by BioCosmetic Research Labs says that some AHA's are, *"...derived from sugar cane,"* and is a, *"Natural acid that tends to give an exfoliating property where it keeps the pores open, smooth the skin, and smooth the texture."* But most importantly to the consumer using the product, Dr. Burgess says fulfills the desire of people wanting to keep their skin looking youthful. Dr. Burgess admits, *"I use them and I love them, and most people who do really like them."*

AHA's are non-toxic, natural acids found in sour milk (lactic acid), apples and apple juice (malic acid), sugar cane (glycolic acid), citrus fruits (citric acid) and grapes or wine (tartaric acid). AHA's are not new says Dr. Burgess, it's known that Mary Queen of Scots use to soak in red wine to renew her youthful appearance. But modern day remedies have sophisticated themselves in lotions and creams.

Dr. Burgess purports that some of the AHA products are, *"...used over the counter, most of them are used in a physician's office for chemical peeling. But over the counter the most popular is Glycolic acid. The majority of them that are over the counter are very low in percentage, which most people don't realize."* AHA's as with all other cosmetic ingredients are regulated by the FDA (Food and Drug Administration). The strength of AHA-based products range between 1 to 2% for most department and drugstore products, up to as high as 80% used by doctors only.

The use of alpha hydroxy acid in over the counter products began in 1990 when Origins introduced it in their face cream Starting Over, followed immediately by Avon's Anew, Estee Lauder's Fruition, La Prairie's Age Management Serum (which contains 5% of lactic acid) and Revlon's Results. Since then, a profusion of alpha hydroxy acid products have bombarded the marketplace. Use of the ingredient causes some skin to flake and feel itchy. Dr. Burgess response is, *"If there's a little bit of flakiness, that is the skin sloughing, which is what its suppose to do. If you feel grit or crumbles, its probably something in the product itself, you should not feel a grit on your face, you should get a very light peeling, very similar to dandruff."* These side effects, along with a slight stinging should last only after a week of use.

Generating cell renewal, AHA products plump up your skin's dermis layer by sloughing off or exfoliating the outermost layer (stratum corneum) of your skin. Although your skin normally exfoliates itself every 30 days by generating a new outer layer of skin, Dr. Burgess says the extra help that alpha hydroxy acids offer can only provide more efficient cell turnover. *"It keeps the skin more active,"* Dr. Burgess explains.

"When you use a washcloth, you are exfoliating; when you dry yourself with a towel, you're exfoliating faster. In a sense [using AHA's], you're just getting those dead cell layers off a little bit sooner than them just falling off naturally. And the more the cell falls off the top, the more it generates and stimulates the development at the bottom through that 30-day cycle."

Alpha hydroxy acids are also said to be good humectants (moisture-magnets), because they allow the skin to drink-in more moisture by slightly stripping the skin of dead cell layers. AHA's also work well on sun damaged skin, reducing photo-aging, which is the breakdown of elastin and collagen in your skin (the skin's support system), inevitably leading to wrinkly, sagging skin. One would argue that thinning the outer layer of the skin would elicit more damage than not, but in a University of Pennsylvania study, dermatologists reported a 20% thickening in the epidermis after only two weeks of using ammonium lactate (a 12% lactic acid derivative). So in essence, AHA actually assists your skin's natural ability to ward off dirt, pollutants and other environmental aggressions.

Some cosmetic houses like Revlon and Shiseido are even going a step further in AHA efficacy by patenting exclusive ingredients that word in tandem with AHA's, or as a replacement to them altogether. Shiseido uses between 1 and 2% AHA to produce softening and moisturization to the skin.

Bio-EPO and Bio Hyaluronic Acid they say produces even more energizing and moisturizing effects than AHA's alone. Revlon patented MPG (Methoxypropyl Gluconamide), which allows the company not to use AHA in their products at all. MPG is purported to be a neutral, non-acid compound that is prevalent in their Results skin care line, penetrating within the skin's upper layer, minimizing dead cell build-up and helping remove the dry, damaged cells that can clog the facial surface. They say fresher cells can then rise to the surface.

Other products that I recommend containing AHA, or AHA-like properties are: Elizabeth Arden's Ceramide Time Complex Moisture Cream, said to help reduce the appearance of fine lines and wrinkles...and to help fortify and replenish your skin's moisture barrier.

PART 6

MAKEUP FOR THE MINIMALIST: THE CANVAS & THE STORY

FOUNDATION

In art, the first steps in painting a portrait is properly priming the canvas before adding color to tell the story. The same rule can be applied for painting your face with cosmetics. Singer Karyn White says, *"The most important thing to Black women is to make sure [your] foundation matches so you won't have too light of a color, too dark or too red."* Because Karyn is such a stickler for matching her foundation, she finds herself mixing and matching a lot of shades together to find her exact shade. Explains Karyn, *"Because there are so many tones to Black skin, I try to use a foundation that's really close. I use Naomi Simms and sometimes I use Joe Blasco. I also mix a lot of the foundations together to come up with my own color."*

Foundation or bases are designed to make your face look as though you have naturally flawless skin, as if you were wearing no makeup at all. Uneven skin tones, blemishes, birthmarks, oil and shine can all be diffused with a deft application of foundation. New York Makeup Artist Sam Fine is the super-models makeup man of choice. Appointed as one of Revlon's spokesman for their line ColorStyle [a line exclusively for women of color], Sam explains that *"You can do makeup with anything. It's the training and the education that's needed. Women have to understand that makeup doesn't have to be heavy, it's not all cream foundations. We [Revlon] have liquids and oil-free. It's educating women that they can wear anything they want as long as they pick the right colors."*

You can wear foundation over your entire face for a full structured look, or you can target cover, using your base only where you feel its needed most. Some of the more upscale bases on the market are specially designed for this need. Moisturizer/pigment combinations, often referred to as Tint N' Color's, lightly diffuse blemishes and gives your skin a smooth even texture while adding moisture. also protect your skin from environmental radicals that your face endures during the course of your day such as air conditioning, humidity, dry heat, pollution and UV rays. Clarins Moisturizing Tint SPF 6 is a great Tint N' Color to try out if you want a light-weight coverage.

There are basically two formulations of foundations: Liquids and Creams, with modification in between. Liquid foundations are water based formulations that offer the least and lightest amount of coverage and they are best used by oily, combination, and normal skin types. Liquid bases won't clog pores either, whereas some oil based foundations basically layer oil on top of oily skin and eventually lead to blackheads and other skin eruptions.

Cream foundations are a melding of oil, powder and pigment, heavier in coverage and application than that of liquid bases, cream foundations are best used on dryer skin's, which need to retain hydration with an oil base, or for women who want a more defined look to their makeup.

QUICK TIP:

If you want to test your foundation to see whether or not it's an oil base or water base, try this test. Put some of your foundation in a saucer and add a couple of drops of water. If it mixes freely, the base is water-loving or "hydrophilic." If it doesn't mix well, then it's "hydrophobic" or a water hating, oil-based makeup.

QUICK TIP:

If you have dry skin and use a cream based foundation, but prefer the sheerness of a liquid, wet your cosmetic sponge (found in drugstores) before applying your cream base then apply as normal. The water in the sponge will help thin the coverage consistency.

QUICK TIP:

The best way to test any foundation or base shade for your skin tone is first testing it on your collarbone or jawline. Never test a base shade for color accuracy on the back of your hand, or on the inside of your wrist, due to the fact that the skin color on your hands and wrists are much lighter than the actual skin color on your face. This could have you choosing a shade of foundation that is two or three shades lighter than your actual skin color.

APPLICATION: Foundation

a) Apply a dab of foundation on your cosmetic sponge and quickly apply to the five motor points of your face. (nose, chin, center of forehead and both cheeks).

b) Once applied, blend foundation using upward and outward motions to relieve your skin of gravity, which can pull and cause sagging and premature wrinkling.

c) BLEND, BLEND, BLEND!

The most important three words you should remember whenever applying foundation is BLEND, BLEND, BLEND! Makeup Artist Deborah Lake, who has worked for the recording artist formally known as Prince and several other mega-stars explains, *"I make people look very natural. I truly believe that the face is my canvas, so I want to perfect it as beautifully as I can. My greatest asset is that I can blend very well. It's an internal gift with being able to match up the best foundation and powders, because when you start with that, everything else seems to fall in line."* Rolonda Watts also believes in the Blend, Blend, Blend motto. She admits, *"I'm learning that less is best. As I'm getting older, I'm knowing that the more you put on the older you look."*

To make certain that your base is thoroughly blended, take your sponge and use a technique derived from facial massage called "tapotement"-a light tapping movement that is used to blend foundation. This technique removes the appearance of uneven lines and demarcation and also aids the heavy-handed who may be applying too much foundation and need to spread their foundation thinly over the skin.

QUICK TIP:

To preset your foundation before or after powder, take some Aveda's Toning/Firming Mist and spritz your face with it. After which, take a tissue, wrap it around your cosmetic sponge and lightly blot your skin. This technique will further blend your foundation by removing any excess oil and base build-up.

In my last interview with the late, soul songstress Vesta, she shared with me a unique way of setting her makeup in the morning. She says after applying her foundation and powder, she sits in her shower and allows the steam to moisture-set her canvas.

SPECIAL QUICK TIP: Matching foundation undertones for women of color

For most women of color, including Native American, Hispanic, Asian, Indian, African, African-American and Middle Eastern, they have a yellow undertone to their skin as opposed to the pink and red undertones that was suggested by many of the older cosmetic companies.

One line that has literally swept the cosmetic buying country off its feet is Iman Cosmetics. A line exclusively designed to address the foundation needs of all women of color. Since there are about 36 different classifications of African American skin tones, Iman's Second To None Cream Powder Foundation comes in 16 shades, all blended with yellow and gold undertones to match every skin tone. *"I go to cosmetic counters and buy three, four foundations and go home and mix and match-why do I have to do that? It's insulting for a consumer to have to do this,"* Iman insists.

Iman's foundations offers women of color the coverage and spreadability of a cream and the velvety finish of a powder with a soft, matte finish. These shades are divided into three categories for simplicity: Sand (1-5), Clay (1-5) and Earth (1-5) -- all accommodating light, medium and dark ranges. Iman says, *"I have a real sensitivity to who the true women of color is. She is not merely one ethnic group; she is African American, Hispanic, Asian American and Native American. I believe that women of color, are the women of the world."* Iman points out that, *"It's time to address the concerns of this invisible consumer because today's minorities are tomorrow's majority."*

Her Luxury Pressed Powder is talc-free and comes in six shades to perfectly match the undertones of the foundations. Formulated without frost or mica, it has the properties of a loose powder when applied with a brush. It too uses the same easy to understand categories, Sand (Light and Light-Medium), Clay (Medium and Medium-Dark) and Earth (Dark and Deep).

And since women of color have a constant battle with shine-through during the course of a day, Iman also developed an Under Cover Agent Oil Control Lotion to refine texture and dispel shine. Topped with her Corrective Concealer-six shades to compliment the Sand, Clay and Earth categories-the foundation system is most complete.

CONCEALER

You know that puffiness under your eyes? Those dark circles that sleep won't dispel? Well, they're technically called Chloasma, but they are ruthlessly referred to as "bags!"

To conceal or not to conceal...there is no question! If you have bothersome skin flaws and under eye circles that you can't stand, don't procrastinate...hide it! Having dark circles under your eyes, skin blemishes or minor birthmarks on your face, are tell-tale arrows that point in the direction of a face needing to go under cover. You may not have been born with perfect skin, but that doesn't mean you have to live with it!

Facial flaws are not to be seen and luckily, there are a number of effective concealers in today's marketplace that offer secret agent concealment with total undercover benefits. Under eye concealer or camouflage cream come in stick and pot form and should only be one or two shades lighter than your foundation. If camouflage cream is too light, you could end up looking like a raccoon. And subsequently, if your concealer is too dark, you'll defeat the entire purpose of using it in the first place.

In some cases, women don't necessarily need to wear a foundation at all, and only need to wear an under eye concealer. If your skin tone is somewhat even and unblemished, then this rule definitely applies. However, if you prefer to wear both, it's important not to apply too much. Concealer is usually a thicker, heavier version of a foundation. When concealer, foundation and powder are layered together, if not blended well, the visual result can be disastrous.

Concealers of late have gotten to be very sophisticated. The newer brands of concealer diffuse light and provides a smooth, even skin appearance. In order for concealers to have that light-diffusing quality, cosmetic houses have added powder-fine titanium dioxide, silica and mica flakes to some of their concealers.

One of the best and most popular concealers on the market is the critically acclaimed Dermablend by Flori Roberts. Derma Blend comes in 9 cover cream shades and can be blended to match the palest of ivory to the deepest of ebony skin's. Coupled with a sheer, waterproof, translucent powder to conceal, Dermablend reveals a true-to-life skin that is impeccable to the naked eye.

APPLICATION: Concealer

a) Take a thin dab of concealer on your fingertips or, flat brush and apply just under each eye, right in the crest of the circle.

b) Using a clean sponge applicator, use the touch and press, tapotement movement to blend and thin out concealer in a half moon shape.

c) Now take a small dab of your foundation applied to your sponge and very gently dab around the edges where the concealer ends. This technique gives an imperceptible look to your overall canvas.

QUICK TIP:

Unless you are an entertainer under harsh stage lighting, or have a severe case of chloasma [dark under eye circles], never use lavender, mint green or white concealers under your eyes-the look is too harsh and most difficult to blend.

QUICK TIP:

If you're in a rush and find you're plum out of concealer, instead you can use a foundation one to two shades lighter than the actual foundation you normally use.

POWDER

Now that your foundation and concealer is applied, it's time to seal and set your face, giving your skin a no-shine, matte finish using translucent sealer or face powder. Face powder is the final step in preparing the canvas. A lot of women think that translucent means one color that works for everyone, but that's not the case. Translucent powders come in many shades, although most companies have only a few basics. If a cosmetics company doesn't have a translucent sealer to match your skin perfectly, shop around, or try using baby powder.

Baby powder you say? Yes, baby powder! Most commercial loose and pressed powders are made from talc, a mined mineral that's actually a form of crushed marble. You can hardly see it on the skin once it has been allowed to set. If you were to look under a microscope, you would see that talc is composed of little fine plates that lie flat, coating your skin with a silky layer, making your skin feel smooth. Titanium or mica are also added to face powders to make the talc opaque, the color is mixed in via iron oxides like burnt sienna, burnt umber and ferric oxide, creating light, medium and dark powders.

There are basically two kinds of face powders: 1) Loose translucent powder and 2) Pressed translucent powder. Loose powder is used to set the final application of foundation, while Pressed powder is used mostly to touch-up your makeup when applicable.

Cosmetic companies have as many face powders as they do foundations, but all face powders do basically the same thing-set your foundation and give your skin a matte finish. Although there are face powders formulated in lighter weights and textures, many other face powders are heavier in weight for stronger oil absorption. This accounts for many women's makeup to have a heavy, caked-on appearance. Also some face powders are very rich in pigment and may cause your foundation to change color and appear artificial.

APPLICATION: Powder

a) Using a clean cosmetic sponge, take your loose powder in the palm of your hand and press sponge into powdered palm.

b) Now press powder over your entire face, until there are no hotspots or shining areas.

c) A lot of women prefer to use a large Fluff brush to apply their face powder. I've realized that some, but not all, Fluff brushes are made equal. Some can streak your foundation and leave small lines and brush hairs across your face, causing an unfinished look.

d) To avoid this possible dilemma, pressing loose powder on your face works to set your foundation quicker and more thoroughly.

e) After which, take a spritz of Evian Water or Mineral Mist spray your face lightly.

f) Then take the unused side of your sponge and begin a technique called "Buffing" or "Smoothing." Buff your face in short, downward strokes beginning from your forehead, ending under your chin and decollage, so that the fine hairs that cover your face will lay flat on the surface of your skin, creating a matte appearance.

g) This technique will ensure a smooth, long lasting powder/foundation blend and application.

h) You should continue this Buffing technique until all excess powder has been removed and your face has a matte, even texture to it. Now you're ready for color!

SPECIAL QUICK TIP: Cosmetic Brushes

As aforementioned, many women prefer using brushes as opposed to cosmetic sponges. For easy use and quality application, here are the brushes I recommend. M.A.C. Hand Sculpted Brushes (800)

387-6707. Ilise Heitzner Harris Cosmetic Art Brushes (212) 594-8253. Bobbi Brown Essentials Travel Brush Set or Deluxe Brush Set (212) 753-9500. Call for free brochures and literature.

QUICK TIP:

If you use expensive brushes to apply your makeup, proper cleansing and care of your brushes is most important. En Vogue's Makeup Artist Troy Jensen says, *"I clean my brushes with a combination of baby shampoo and witch hazel. Then I rinse them with a little bit of conditioner, and then lay them on a towel to air dry overnight."* He prefers to use Sable and Squirrel-haired brushes.

QUICK TIP:

Some women feel there is no need to wear foundation all of the time, and prefer to wear just a loose or pressed powder like natural beauties, actress, Karyn Parsons and singer, Karyn White. If this describes you, apply a small dab of concealer under your eyes, blend, and press powder gently on the skin. End your blending with the "Smoothing" movement.

IN YOUR FACE - COLOR HARMONY

Telling Your Story With Color

Once you've primed your canvas and harnessed your theme for the day, now it's time to tell your story using the cosmetic colors of eyeshadow, cheek color, and lip color. There are no hard and fast rules when coordinating cosmetic colors, its an individual expression and art. Some women prefer to wear monochromatic colors, a look that wears with almost any wardrobe styling, whereas other women wear almost no makeup color at all, getting by with just eyeliner, mascara and maybe a tint of lip color. Soul singer, Cherrelle is one of those women. *"I'm not a makeup girl, she professes. "I am so subdued you would not believe. I do like Makeup Artist's to make me look pretty, that's when the little girl in me comes out and that's when I feel I look pretty when they make me up to look like the girls in the books."*

Of course there are those who would never think about leaving the house if their lipstick, nail polish, blush and eyeshadow were not color coordinated. Vesta exclaimed, *"I will go to hell and high water to find a lipstick, nail polish and toenail polish that is the exact same shade! Because I'm constantly getting manicures and pedicures!"* In my last interview with the late songstress Phyllis Hyman. She said, *"Some entertainers deliberately wear no makeup. Oh no, that's not my ticket at all! I like being glamorous, I like dressing up, wearing makeup, putting on hats and nice clothes."*

Nonetheless, in order to tell a story with color, you should have a basic understanding of color harmony and what colors blend best with others and compliment your skintone. But most importantly, for women on the go, the application should be quick, simple and efficient. Gone are the days where women have the time to spend hours on lengthy makeup preparations, simplicity is the key objective.

Learning what shades, colors and hues are right for you can profoundly impact the way you look and feel about yourself. For example, bright colors like reds, yellows and vibrant pinks express a dramatic, self-confident personality type, impressing joy and excitement. Darker, more neutral/natural shades like dark taupes, grays, rusts, browns and moody blues give the impression of subtle freshness.

The object of the game is not to spend a lot of your time finding the makeup hues that present the liveliest and truest expression of yourself, but more so, developing an attitude that will cause you to shine regardless of what combination of colors you choose to wear. Always remember, you wear the makeup, the makeup does not wear you!

Makeup Artist and Creative Director for Iman Cosmetics Byron Barnes shares a similar viewpoint about simplifying color. He says, *"My approach to makeup is-I call it the 'Three C's': Uncontrived, Unconstructed and Uncomplicated. I never want it to look like architecture. I don't want women to be harsh when I do their faces. I'm really big on what I call color harmonies. A lot of women have color wars existing on their face-the color intensity of the blush is too much or she has blue-red lipstick on and brown blusher and pink eyeshadow."*

Byron's goal when designing a face he says is to bring, "A color harmony for eyes, lips, and cheeks that is all within similar color intensity and tonality. I might do all browns, or all plums and mauves, but all of the colors are all in the same color ranges." With Byron's philosophy, all the woman on the move needs to know is the basics of color harmony.

What Is Color Harmony

There are basically two categories of colors with Neutral as an optional third. To make color harmony easy to understand lets break down the basic structure of these three categories. Warm colors are defined as any hues that are yellow based such as: Browns, tans, golds, light greens, oranges, and reds. Cool colors are hues that are blue based like: Pinks, fuchsias, purples, dark greens, plums and lavenders. Neutral colors are shades of black and white like slate grays and charcoal grays that can be blended with warm and/or cool colors, allowing a color to become lighter or darker without changing its primary hue.

For example, if you were to take a shade of tan eyeshadow and add gray, it would turn into a darker brown. The color is still the same, its just been slightly neutralized with the combination of black and white to create a grayish dark brown.

To test color harmony combinations, I suggest taking the Color Harmony Facial Chart, featured on the next page, make copies and apply actual cosmetic colors suggested in this book on the chart. By playing with various color combinations, it will help you personalize and design a variety of facial wardrobes to compliment your dress attire, mood and motive.

Do one chart using warm colors and then do another chart using cool colors, then take your finished Facial Chart and harmonize your wardrobe colors with the dominant colors on your facial chart.

Philippe Matthews

COLOR HARMONY CHART

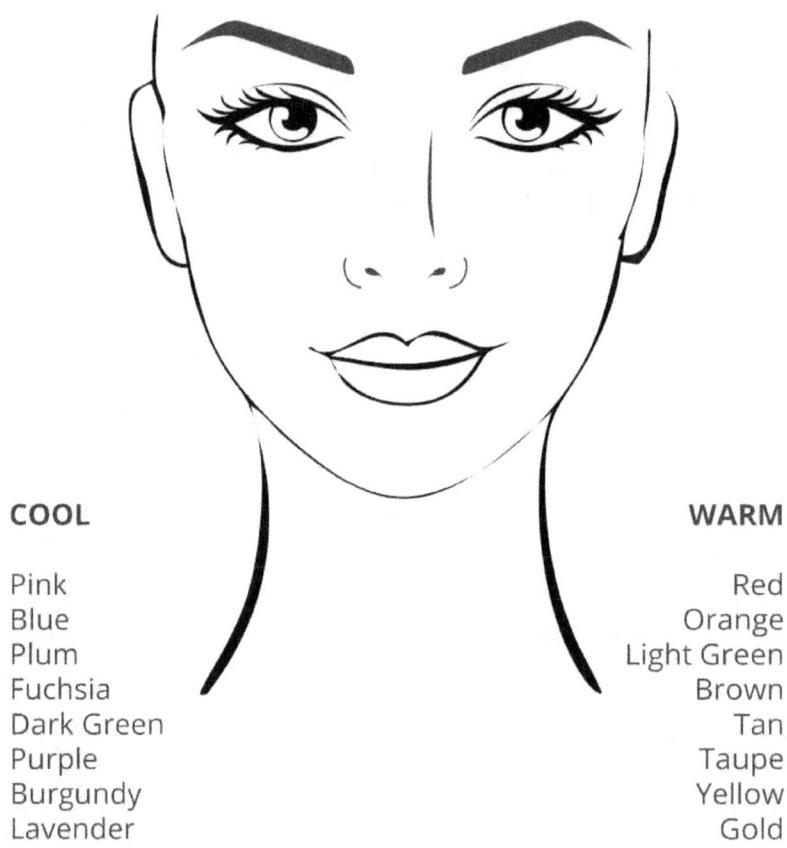

COOL

Pink
Blue
Plum
Fuchsia
Dark Green
Purple
Burgundy
Lavender

WARM

Red
Orange
Light Green
Brown
Tan
Taupe
Yellow
Gold

QUICK TIP:

Take the Color Harmony Facial Chart and draw a vertical line from forehead to chin, splitting the face into two halves. Label the left side Cool and the right side Warm, then color each side using the respective cosmetic colors. When shopping for wardrobe selection, you can then use this Color Harmony Facial Chart as a guide to choosing and designing your own personal makeup image.

Now that you have a basic understanding of color harmony, let's look at creating an actual color story beginning with the windows of the soul-your eyes. I'm going to focus on a simple day makeup theme. Something that's simple, quick and should take you all of five minutes to apply once you've mastered the basics.

• *EYELINER*

Regardless of how much eyeshadow a woman may wear, nothing sets off a beautiful pair of eyes better than eyeliner. The first and most important step in eye defining is learning the proper usage of Eyeliner.

Eyeliner creates depth and dimension for your eyes, making them appear larger and more alive. Plus, it gives the illusion of lush, plush lashes, even where there may not be any lashes at all. For day wear, brown, charcoal gray or midnight blue colors work well.

APPLICATION: Eyeliner

a) When lining, make sure you get as close to your top lash-line as possible, ensuring a natural look.

b) Start at the inner corner of your eye and line outward.

c) There are many different ways in which you can use liner to emphasize or de-emphasize the size of your eyes. Whether you line the top lid of your eyes only, the entire rim of your eye, or a half circle on the outer corners, it's an individual choice that will be decided on the type of lifestyle, personality, and purpose of your day.

QUICK TIP:

Makeup Artist for Prince, Deborah Lake avows, "*I don't use a lot of pencils around the eyes, I use more eyeshadows. I've learned to use makeup shadows and brushes in place of a pencil, so I do a lot of my shading and lining with an angled brush and powder eyeshadow.*"

Philippe Matthews

QUICK TIP:

Eyeliner worn on the rim of the lower lid next to the eye often leads to infection and is not advisable. Also, by lining the inner rim of your eye makes your eyes appear smaller, rather than larger.

If you do line the inner rim of your eyes, or if you use a lot of eye makeup, always use a good eye makeup remover. Janet Sartin's Gentle Eye Makeup Remover Pads are excellent.

• *BROWS*

If someone were to ask you-aesthetically speaking, what were the most pronounced lines of expression on your face? Chances are you'd likely answer, *"My eyebrows."* The eyebrow in technical talk is really supposed to just keep dust and debris from falling into your eyes, but the brow is capable of much more than that. The brow can produce expressions of seduction and allure, joy and happiness, or sorrow and dismay without the utterance of a single word.

The brows have gone through a vast montage of styles and trends throughout the decades. They've been penciled in, pulled and plucked out. From the drawn-on lines of Jean Harlow and Dorothy Dandridge to the deep stages of Elizabeth Taylor and Audrey Hepburn. We even went through a bushy decade with the wild and woolly Brooke Shields.

Brows no longer have to set facial trends by being bushy, or thin and tweezed to no end. The new brow has its own reality and individuality. If you wear your brows naturally arched and soft-spoken-keeping the brow hairs to a minimum and remembering to fill in any areas where the hairs may be sparse, you'll forever be in trend.

Whenever applying color to the brows, make sure to always follow the natural arch in which your brow grows. Use a dark brown or charcoal gray, matte powder, instead of an eyeliner pencil for a softer, more natural look.

APPLICATION: *Brows*

a) Using an angled brush or a Q-tip, apply a small amount of brow color on wand or brush and begin applying color on the inner corners of your brows outward until the desired shape and density has been reached.

b) If you apply too much brown color, take a clean Q-tip and remove excess with a light moisturizer.

QUICK TIP:

To train your eyebrows, before going to bed, apply a thick coat of petroleum jelly to them. Then brush your brows with a brow brush or a clean toothbrush in the direction that you wish for them to grow. After a few weeks of this browbeating, you should notice a new growth direction in your brows.

QUICK TIP:

You can also try taming your brows with one of the oldest makeup tricks in the books. Take a defunct tooth brush, lace it with super-hold hair spray, and brush your brows in whatever direction you feel fit before beginning your day.

• *MASCARA*

They say beauty is in the eyes of the beholder. Well behold, the eyes reveal the deepest emotions of the soul, and the epitome of eye allure can be best identified by the bat of a lash, or a wink of an eye. Flattering, fluttering eyelashes help express a woman's mystery and sensuality even if a woman wears falsies behind a pair of glasses it still lends itself to the glamorous glances of legendary lash lovers like Lena Horne, Dorothy Dandridge, Diana Ross, Pearl Bailey, and Diahann Carroll.

After you've applied your eyeliner, you should use mascara to lengthen, thicken and stretch your lashes. A good mascara won't cake or clump your lashes together, or cause your lashes to dehydrate. Brown, black and blue mascara's are the recommended colors for the most natural look.

It is estimated that 90 percent of women in America wear mascara, even if they do not wear any other kind of makeup. Some women purchase their mascara in department stores, but the majority of women (80%), purchase their mascara in drugstores. It was reported in a fashion magazine that for 15 years the number one selling mascara of choice by women has been Maybelline's Great Lash Mascara in the pink and green tube. They report selling one mascara every two seconds!

APPLICATION: Mascara

a) Using the tip of the mascara wand, held in a vertical position, stroke mascara on the tips of your lashes to apply color.

b) Then with the flat of the wand, held in a horizontal position, brush lashes in an upward, zig zagging motion to separate.

QUICK TIP:

A neat trick to speed up your morning color process is to take a little mascara from your wand and whisk it over your eyebrows to fill in sparse areas, giving them shape and definition.

QUICK TIP:

Mascara is quick to dry out before its been used up, so don't pump your mascara wand in and out of the container. When you do this, you let in air, causing the mascara to dry out. Instead, as you pull the mascara wand out, slowly twirl it around inside the tube so it's fully coated with mascara when removed, then apply.

QUICK TIP:

Failing to thoroughly remove eye makeup, especially mascara, each night can clog up the hair follicle on the eyelids, leading to infection. So make sure to cleanse lashes of mascara using proper eye makeup remover. Remember Janet Sartin's Gentle Eye Makeup Remover Pads are one of the best.

Eyeliner, mascara and brow color offer the frame for the color story of the eyeshadow you'll be using. Now let's find a shade of eyeshadow that will best compliment an active day look.

• *EYESHADOW*

Classic beauty can always be defined by classic eyes; eyes that are not overly made up, but subtly enhanced to show depth, dimension and natural contour. A man who put the class in beauty and spearheaded many of the classic trends and beauty styles for other Makeup Artist's to follow is the legendary Joey Mills.

His career has spanned more than twenty years, and he's designed such alluring eyes as: Diana Ross, Lena Horne, Liza Minelli and Cicely Tyson to Princess Caroline, Camile Cosby, Whitney Houston, Grace Jones and Barbara Walters. His classic makeup and eye designs have graced over 800 magazine covers worldwide, and his million dollar techniques were immortalized in his bestselling book New Classic Beauty.

Joey says many makeup styles have come and gone, but the classic face will always have longevity. *"The classic look will never change,"* he states. *"But what has changed is that we have more women of different colors wanting that classic look, which means color is much more important in makeup now. What I've done is brought wonderful colors to women so they can make that look easier."*

The Joey Mills System is a line of mini-cosmetic and lip color kits, specifically designed for travel, quick touch-ups and no frills beauty. The kits were designed to cover the entire complexion spectrum. Ivory is recommended for lighter, fair-skinned women such as blondes and brunettes, Tawny defines the medium skin tone range for Asians and Hispanics, and Bronze and Mahogany cover the richest complexions ranges of women of color, such as African-American and Native American women. These three kits bring class and definition to the entire face-especially the eyes.

Each kit contains a total of ten compact eyeshadows to choose from that fit neatly into a travel bag or purse, and is supported of course with two blushers, a tube of mascara, two corrector colors, a mini-foundation and finishing powder. In designing the line Joey says, *"I pulled from the fifteen years that I worked with Calvin Klein, Ralph Lauren and Bill Blass."*

Philippe Matthews

Joey says he also pulled his ideas from his experiences of working the London, Italy, Paris and Rome couture shows with fashion cartels Versace, Valentino, Chanel and Yves Saint Laurent. *"I did them every three months! I had to develop different colors, because I had to go from blonde to Iman, and this was one show of fifteen to twenty girls! I had to stay up all night and mix colors, and darken them and tint them. So with all those years of experience, I just learned."*

No woman can hide her true emotions behind her sensuality of sight. Songstress Ce Ce Peniston says that her eyes talk regardless of what mood she's in. *"They talk when I'm happy, they talk when I'm sad, they talk when I'm glowing. My eyes speak for me no matter what mood I'm in. I can smile all want to, but my eyes will tell on me."*

You don't need to saturate your lids with four or more shades of color in order to create drama, depth and allure. Even though, a collection of concentrated colors may give an optical illusion of ocular compliment, there is no need for an eyelid to be full of matte, frost and super-frost eyeshadows fighting for identification. Proactive women understand the philosophy that less is more.

Joey shared a story with me that gets to the point of less is more when it comes to pulsating a woman's pupils. *"Not too long ago while working at Valentino in Rome with photographer* Patrick Demarchilier,*"* Joey explains, *"Beverly [Johnson] and I were having a problem doing a beauty cover shot for Italian Bazaar. We were asked to come up with an attitude which, while wearing a hat, would communicate beauty and sophistication starting with an everyday American look. Basically we needed to go from plain to glamorous. We both realized how much the eyes are the windows to the soul and grasping that idea in the shot became the way to succeed."*

JOEY'S QUICK TIP:

"Your main beauty ritual is to always try to add a soft expression which relates to family, friends and work associates. This expression even for the totally makeup free woman comes from the eye area. You want to concentrate on easy, quick eye makeup

focusing on eye brows and eyeshadow contour keeping it all within a very natural look. This is how you add a soft sparkle and glow to your expression without overdoing it. You should have total awareness of your skin tone and complexion with emphasis on how specific colors affect the warmth of your skin. You want to recognize the difference between the ivory, bronze, tawny tan, olive and mahogany tones in you skin so you can choose colors which compliment your skin tones. For eyeglass wearers, be advised that you may have to emphasize the depth of color and toned to compensate for the glasses. Be sure to wear glasses which are a genuine fashion accessory paying careful attention to shape and style of frames; they act the same as eye makeup."

There are many eye colors and textures for you to choose from on the market. Mattes, of course, wear the longest and offer the most natural look, while frosts and semi-frosts are used primarily to add drama, highlight and attention. Some women wear eyeshadows for a look of seduction, some wear it for the illusion of a brighter expression. Others may wear eyeshadow the way they saw their mother wearing it twenty years ago, and some women insist on not wearing any at all. All and all, choosing an eyeshadow palette is a very intimate session indeed.

A general rule of thumb though in choosing proper eye shades is using the dominant colors of your wardrobe as a guide to selecting a complementary eyeshadow palette. So let's assume for a moment that your wardrobe is predominantly corporate America, with neutral shades of gray, navy blue, and brown being the main hue. If these are the dominant colors in your closet, stick with taupes, rusts, deep golds, light browns and oranges, burnt siennas in your eyeshadow selection. But remember, you can always use the Color Harmony Facial Chart to make the best selection.

APPLICATION: Eyeshadow

a) For a soft day look with attitude, select two matte shades of eye color, a light and a dark.

b) Take an eyeshadow applicator or baby fluff brush and sweep one of the shades you chose in your Color Harmony Face Chart across your entire lid and eye area for even color saturation.

c) Then with a shade of charcoal gray or dark brown eyeshadow, add to the lids and crease of your eyes.

d) Take a Q-tip to fade the line of the darker shadow to reduce harshness of edges.

QUICK TIP:

If you're in a hurry woman and only want a dab of color, take dab of blusher and sweep it over your eyelids, crease and brow bone.

QUICK TIP:

Another great trick for blending your eyeshadow is taking a dab of loose powder and whisking it over your eyes with a brush or cosmetic sponge. This technique will also help set the eyeshadow and allow the color to last longer.

• *BLUSH*

Everyone knows what it feels like to blush. A sensation of warmth, of blood rushing to the surface of your skin, spreads from your neck all over your face. In choosing a blush, use one that compliments your skin tone. For example, if your skin tone is more yellow, use a cheek color in the russet, brown, taupe or deep orange family (Warm based). If your skin is pinkish or bluish in tone, use cheek colors in the pink, plum and burgundy family (Cool based). Using this rule of thumb when selecting cheek color will always give your face balance. Again, use the Color Harmony Face Chart for accuracy.

BYRON BARNES QUICK TIP:

Byron Barnes explained his advice for cheek sleeks, saying, *"I'm very light-handed. I like to do blusher very light-hit-it and quit-it. Its part of your complexion, and it should never have the impact that eyes and lips have."*

APPLICATION: Blush

a) With the color of your choice, apply cheek color lightly to the apple of your cheeks with a cosmetic sponge or blush brush.

b) Blend upward and outward toward your temples.

QUICK TIP:

If you've found that you have over applied your cheek color, use the same technique that was described in the Quick Tip for blending your eyeshadow. Take a dab of loose powder and brush it over your cheeks to soften the edges.

• LIP COLOR

Whether you wear bold shades or subtle shades, lip color makes a statement that can change the entire look of your face, or even influence your personality in a matter of seconds. A woman's lips can say so much, long before a single syllable has ever been uttered. The trick to obtaining the perfect pout is not necessarily the color you choose, but in the way you choose to use it.

Start by selecting a shade that is color compatible with the dominant hue in your eyeshadows, i.e., if your eyeshadow and wardrobe is yellow based or Warm, use lip colors in the red, coral, brown, bronze, gold, and orange family. Likewise, if your eyeshadow and wardrobe is blue based or Cool, use lip colors that are in the burgundy, plum, pink, fuchsia, and watermelon family.

Actress Karyn Parsons explains her favorite lip color is red. *"I love wearing red lipstick. I've been using Clinique Different Lipstick Ripe Raisin lip color and Super Spice. They also have an Earth Red that's really nice. I've been told by other makeup artists that I have a wonderful mouth, so when I make up my face, that's where I focus most of my attention."*

Ce Ce Peniston says, *"Red looks good on my lips, browns and sometimes pink, but usually I'll stick with browns and rose colors."*

JOEY MILLS QUICK TIP:

Joey Mills says the most natural and best colors for lips are, *"True reds, burgundies, purples and maroons."* His application advice is to *"Use a lip pencil or lip brush to create a color contoured lip line and fill in with lipstick or pencil color. A pencil is also excellent as all over mouth color and as a semi-permanent base for lipstick. If using a darker liner shade, be sure to blend into the lighter color for a smooth look."*

Generally, there are four categories of lip colors to choose from: Matte, semi-matte, frost and creams. Matte and semi-matte lip colors have always offered the strongest and longest wear in terms of texture and stain, although matte lip colors can be drying due to their lack of hydration, many newer formulations contain moisturizing emollients to keep lips moist. Frost and creams offer a brighter, smoother texture with moisture and shine, but may not last as long as matte and semi-matte formulations.

APPLICATION: Lip Color

a) If you're using a semi-matte/matte lip color, then line your lips, using a lip brush, with the actual lip color as opposed to a pencil liner. Matte formulations tend not to bleed, eradicating the need for pencil liner altogether.

b) But if you're using a creme lip color then lip liner should be used.

c) Begin applying lip color in the center of your lips using a lip brush for maximum control, and work your way out to the edges.

QUICK TIP:

To ensure the longest lasting lip stain, try dabbing your lips with 1) foundation, then 2) add powder to set the foundation and 3) apply lip color. After applying lip color, 4) take a thin layer of facial tissue and press over your lips, then 5) take a cosmetic sponge lightly laced with pressed or loose powder and 6) gently press onto the thin layer of facial tissue over your lips. This technique will extend the wear of your lip color, as well as reinforce matte texture.

If your lips are prone to drying in the usage of matte lip colors, dot your lips with a lip moisturizer like Natural Glow's Lip Balm before applying foundation, powder and color.

QUICK TIP:

If you're really in a hurry to get out the door in the morning, taking time to apply foundation, powder and lip color may take up more time than you really have. A technique used often is purchasing lip pencils in the shades of your favorite lip colors and staining your lips with the lip pencil, simply by applying color over your entire lip. A dab of lip gloss and you're off!

QUICK TIP:

If you don't like the taste of most lip colors, most women don't, then try a flavored lip balm like Aveda's aromatherapy Natural Lip Colours their lip colors are an alchemy of plant and flower essences, and are scented and flavored with peppermint and cinnamon that not only tingles on your lips, but help freshen your breath as well!

EPILOGUE

THE JOURNEY COMES TO AN END

Every chapter in this book served as a personal journey. In the beginning, you learned about taking control of your inner thoughts and emotions as a way to deal with the rest of the day. This then progressed slowly into highlighting your outer beauty as a way to make you feel more confident about yourself. Having a well-balanced outlook – both inner and outer – is a key into overcoming any stressful situation you might encounter in any given day.

Yes, the life of a mother is a very hard path to take, but it is one that you should relish in. There's no better feeling in the world knowing that you raised good children and have served your company to the best of your abilities. However, it is quite understandable that the pressures of motherhood, along with work and other external forces might be so hard upon you.

This was a big part as to why this book was created: to show mothers everywhere that you can succeed over stress. Every role that is thrust upon you – mother, wife, employee, boss, sister, daughter, etc – is a role you should cherish and learn to balance well so as not to overwhelm yourself. And this is what this book showed you: that there is always a way to still feel better and look fabulous despite the ever increasing pressures of living in these times.

Chapter Breakdown

In Chapter I, you were introduced to how to start your day on the right foot. Your mood when you wake up dictates what transpires the rest of they day. Even though you know that you will have a stressful day ahead, it's best if you don't think about it that way. All of these negative feelings can be quickly remedied through the power of meditation. Everything from differentiating meditation from prayer to creating a meditative atmosphere are detailed. You even get a special section on tension, relaxation and breath control as these are integral elements to a successful meditative mood. The first chapter also stressed the importance of having a daily ritual just to calm yourself before the stress of work takes over. Basically, it establishes the essence of of having a little "me time" before proceeding to attack the rest of the agenda for the entire day.

The second chapter illustrated the importance of visualization to start the day. By simply visualizing your entire day, you already have this notion deep within you of how the day is going to be. By doing this, you have a sort of inner peace that you can retreat to just in case things get really hectic during the day. You can think of visualizing as a way to release the preordained stresses of the day. The second chapter focused on differentiating visualization from daydreaming. While both may be somewhat the same, there are technical differences between them as visualization is more of an emotional thing. In Chapter II, I provide tips on how you can create an inner sanctuary that will serve as the place you can go to whenever you feel really pressured during the day. This will be your sort-of "happy place" where you can temporarily forget the negative and focus on the positive. The chapter also touches upon the combination of visualization, meditation and exercise.

Chapter III still continued on the theme of developing inner peace, but this time it had a focus on one thing: affirmations. Everybody in this world wants to be assured because this makes them feel more comfortable and gives them more than enough confidence. A tennis player doesn't go out onto the court thinking that she will lose a match because she's up against one of the best players in the entire world. No, she quietly affirms herself of her own strengths and plucks up her courage to give her the confidence that she has a chance to make it. She has a chance to overcome adversity. This is what the third chapter is all about: having affirmations can simply make your day. Not just having affirmations where you can envision peace with a problem, but also personal affirmations. As you continue to recite these to yourself, you will feel a whole lot better about the issues that you have to tackle throughout the day.

In Chapter IV starts quite a journey into the art of putting on makeup. Once you have taken care of what's within, you move on to what's on the outside. Makeup is more than just a girly thing to do. It's something that women can do to make themselves feel much better and give them more than enough confidence to successfully deal with whatever comes their way. With both an internal and external balance, there's no reason why women should feel they couldn't achieve anything. This chapter provides you with the basics of putting on makeup coupled with some relaxation techniques from divas such as Cree Summer, Lisa Fischer and Yolanda Adams. I have also provided my own list of relaxing activities that you can do. These relaxation methods are for you to be calm and clear-headed when you make a decision about how to go about your makeup for the next day. I also provide a guide on taking good care of your skin.

The fifth and last chapter of the book details makeup pointers. This is where you get tips on properly applying foundation, concealer, powder and colors to your face. I stress the value of simplicity and harmony in whatever you choose to paint the canvas with.

I hope that like Alan Cohen in his special message from my SHOCK philosophy book, you have also recognized the power within to make yourself beautiful everyday. *"Reading through these honest and earthy lessons, I was reminded that the principles of success are far simpler than we have been led to believe. The answers, we recognize, are not in complex money-making schemes, but right inside you. Right now, right where you are, you have the genius and talent to magnetize to you all the wealth you desire. And wealth, of course, is far more than just money. Real wealth begins with recognizing your spiritual riches."* And so is real beauty from within.

Parting Words

I sincerely hope you enjoyed this little journey you took on overcoming stress and feeling and looking better through makeup. I hope that the tips and tricks presented here will help you feel a whole lot better when you put them to use.

The life of a mother is one of the most difficult – if not the most difficult – job in the whole world. Hopefully, this book was able to give you some good insights on being able to juggle the many roles that is required of you.

Until then, live life to the fullest and enjoy every moment!

ABOUT THE AUTHOR

Philippe Matthews is a self-empowered, Multi-Media, entrepreneurial maverick. A native of Chicago, Illinois, and former Beauty Editor for Upscale Magazine (1990-1995); Matthews lost both parents as a youth and had to begin working at age 15 to support himself and his older sister. Despite the dire and stressful circumstances of his life, he made good on three promises he made to his mother and did not allow himself to fall prey to the pitfalls in his impoverished community that ensnared so many of his peers. Instead, he forged ahead through life constructively, striving to achieve success and prosperity, developing a powerful and teachable mindset method outlined in: The Shock Wealth System and the Shock Philosophy.

Philippe Matthews is the Executive Director of the HOWmovement.org, a 501c3 dedicated to eliminating Generational Poverty by teaching individuals HOW to MOVE from the illusion of Hope to the Process of HOW, and reveal the potential for success that resides in every child, man and woman. He is also an Internet Marketing Technologist, Book Marketing Shepherd and CEO of MyInternetMarketingExpert.net; an SEO and Social Media Marketing firm near San Francisco.

Philippe is best known as the host of the Philippe Matthews LIVE; a Radio, Internet Video and Blog Show, which has over 1 million collective listeners, viewers and readers worldwide! As a result of Philippe's multimedia internet platform and over 25 years in the business, he has been touted as the "Oprah of Internet" by co-author of Chicken Soup for the Soul, Mark Victor Hansen.

LINKS & RESOURCES:

RECOMMENDED WEBSITES

The HOW Movement
http://www.howmovement.org/

The Philippe Matthews Show
http://www.thepmshow.tv/

My Internet Marketing Expert
http://myinternetmarketingexpert.net/

RECOMMENDED SOCIAL MEDIA SITES

Twitter:
https://twitter.com/thepmshow
https://twitter.com/myiexpert
https://twitter.com/thehowmovement

Facebook:
https://www.facebook.com/thepmshow
https://www.facebook.com/TheHowMovement
https://www.facebook.com/myimexpert

BECOME A PART OF THE HOW MOVEMENT

MISSION STATEMENT

The mission and purpose of the HOW (Helping Ourselves Win) Movement teaches young adults how to empower, educate and train their brains to think like entrepreneurs and social change agents using The Exceptional Rules of Thinking(TM) in order to breakthrough the psychological, emotional, economic and environmental barriers of generational poverty that keep them from reaching their fullest potential.

VISION STATEMENT

The Exceptional Rules of Thinking (TM) has been developed from personal and business life lessons along with in-depth interviews that Philippe Matthews has conducted with world class thought leaders, change agents and experts in the field of human potential. The HOW Movement will produce Internet TV, Radio, and Social Media Content that harnesses the intellectual, emotional and spiritual resources necessary for young adults to live an exceptional life and end the malady of generational poverty.

QUALITY STATEMENT

Learning and deserving to live an exceptional life by training the brain to move from the mindset of why to why not. From victim to victorious. From poverty to wealth. From hope to HOW!

DAILY MANTRA

"I will strive to be exceptional in all I do. Regardless of my birthplace, environment, economic status, family or education; it is my birthright to achieve greatness and live an exceptional life!"

-- Philippe SHOCK Matthews

TAGLINE

Moving from the illusion of Hope to the Process of HOW!

For more than 25 years, I have been researching the psychological effects of poverty and have made some startling connections that have been medically proven. 1) Children born in abject poverty, surrounded by gang violence, verbal/physical abuse, excessive bullying suffer from Severe Depression or PTSD, 2) PTSD weakens and comprises a region of the brain known as the vmPFC "Ventromedial Prefrontal Cortex", 3) A compromised vmPFC creates Learned Helplessness, and 4) Learned Helplessness is the genesis of all addiction and bad habit formation.

This means, we have a society of people "addicted to poverty" because they were born into it and know of no way out! Children who live long enough to survive to see adulthood, suffer from PTSD just like our soldiers coming back from war; only worse. Troops coming back from war once knew what safety was. Kids and adults born in abject poverty and gang violent environments never get to develop that part of their brain that is able to recognize safety and make logical decisions for their future. ! I know this to be true because I am a product of abject poverty and was blessed to be able to get out alive and maintain a benevolent heart but not without severe pain and turmoil however.

I watched both my parents die within two months of each other right before my eyes when I was 14, I was only able to acquire a 6th grade education because I had to stay at home and take care of my mother, I was molested by my alcoholic father, I lived on welfare for years, I worked minimum wage jobs most of my young adult life, I lost all of my possessions and became homeless, I battled (still do) with an eating disorder, went through a crippling betrayal of my marriage that led to divorce and at the same time, I lost a $400,000 lawsuit from an unscrupulous network marketing company with zero dollars in the bank, the list continues!

Now, at age 47, I have lost half my life to the battle of poverty, now I dedicate the rest of my life to eliminating it and training the brains of young people to never have to live the life I have had to endure.

By the grace of God, there go I!

The only reason I did not become a statistic and/or a top news story on CNN is because of three promises I made to my mother which was 1) I will never do drugs, 2) I will never get involved in gang activity and 3) I will make something of my life that you would be proud of.

For decades now, I've been interviewing, studying and learning from the most brilliant minds in the world. Within the last ten years, I have aligned with some of the worlds leading scientists in the field of neuroscience and psychology to produce, develop and disseminate a powerful process to greatly reduce the effects of generational poverty, depression, Learned Helplessness and PTSD at the "brain" level using the HOW Movement's Programs.

OTHER BOOKS BY PHILIPPE SHOCK MATTHEWS:

The Shock Wealth System:
Developing the Mindset to Be Rich Before Becoming Rich

How to Make Millions When Thousands Have Been Laid Off:
Featuring Stedman Graham

The Shock Theology Special Report:
The Dark Side of New Thought Metaphysics & Religious Science

My Four Fathers:
Personal Virtual Interviews with the Worlds Greatest Motivators Who Inspired A Fatherless Son!

S.O.S! - Success Over Stress For the Modern Day Mom in Motion Plus The Motivating Makeover Manual:
Tips, Tricks, and Techniques to Manage Stress & Augment Your Natural Beauty

www.ingramcontent.com/pod-product-compliance
Lightning Source LLC
Chambersburg PA
CBHW070553290526
45790CB00002B/663